Practical Guides in Radiation Oncology

Series editors

Nancy Y. Lee
Department of Radiation Oncology
Memorial Sloan-Kettering Cancer Center
New York, NY, USA

Jiade J. Lu
Department of Radiation Oncology
Shanghai Proton and Heavy Ion Center
Shanghai, China

The series *Practical Guides in Radiation Oncology* is designed to assist radiation oncology residents and practicing radiation oncologists in the application of current techniques in radiation oncology and day-to-day management in clinical practice, i.e., treatment planning. Individual volumes offer clear guidance on contouring in different cancers and present treatment recommendations, including with regard to advanced options such as intensity-modulated radiation therapy (IMRT) and stereotactic body radiation therapy (SBRT). Each volume addresses one particular area of practice and is edited by experts with an outstanding international reputation. Readers will find the series to be an ideal source of up-to-date information on when to apply the various available technologies and how to perform safe treatment planning.

More information about this series at http://www.springer.com/series/13580

Jennifer R. Bellon • Julia S. Wong
Shannon M. MacDonald • Alice Y. Ho
Editors

Radiation Therapy Techniques and Treatment Planning for Breast Cancer

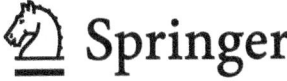 Springer

Editors
Jennifer R. Bellon
Department of Radiation Oncology
Dana-Farber Cancer Institute and Brigham
and Women's Hospital
Harvard Medical School
Boston, Massachusetts
USA

Julia S. Wong
Department of Radiation Oncology
Dana-Farber Cancer Institute and Brigham
and Women's Hospital
Harvard Medical School
Boston, Massachusetts
USA

Shannon M. MacDonald
Department of Radiation Oncology
Massachusetts General Hospital
Harvard Medical School
Boston, Massachusetts
USA

Alice Y. Ho
Department of Radiation Oncology
Memorial Sloan Kettering Cancer Center
New York
USA

Practical Guides in Radiation Oncology
ISBN 978-3-319-40390-8   ISBN 978-3-319-40392-2   (eBook)
DOI 10.1007/978-3-319-40392-2

Library of Congress Control Number: 2016951644

Printed on acid-free paper

This Springer imprint is published by Springer Nature
The registered company is Springer International Publishing AG Switzerland

Contents

Contributors

Estelle Batin, PhD Department of Radiation Oncology,
Francis H Burr Proton Center, Massachusetts General Hospital,
Boston, MA, USA

Carmen Bergom, MD, PhD Department of Radiation Oncology,
Medical College of Wisconsin, Milwaukee, WI, USA

Rachel C. Blitzblau, MD, PhD Department of Radiation Oncology,
Duke University Medical Center, Durham, NC, USA

Oren Cahlon, PhD Department of Radiation Oncology,
Memorial Sloan Kettering Cancer Center, New York, NY, USA

Kimberly S. Corbin Department of Radiation Oncology,
Mayo Clinic, Rochester, MN, USA

Adam Currey, MD Department of Radiation Oncology,
Medical College of Wisconsin, Milwaukee, WI, USA

Nicolas Depauw, PhD Department of Radiation Oncology,
Francis H. Burr Proton Therapy Center, Massachusetts General Hospital,
Boston, MA, USA

Chris J. Diederich, PhD Medical Physics Division,
Department of Radiation Oncology, University of California,
San Francisco, San Francisco, CA, USA

Vishruta Dumane, PhD Department of Radiation Oncology, Icahn School of
Medicine at Mount Sinai, New York, NY, USA

Alice Y. Ho, MD Department of Radiation Oncology, Memorial Sloan Kettering
Cancer Center, New York, NY, USA

Linda Hong, PhD, DABR Department of Medical Physics,
Memorial Sloan Kettering Cancer Center, New York, NY, USA

Kathleen C. Horst, MD Department of Radiation Oncology, Stanford University
School of Medicine, Stanford, CA, USA

Janet K. Horton, MD Department of Radiation Oncology, Duke University Medical Center, Durham, NC, USA

Rachel B. Jimenez, MD Department of Radiation Oncology, Massachusetts General Hospital, Boston, MA, USA

Nataliya Kovalchuk, PhD Department of Radiation Oncology, Stanford University, Stanford, CA, USA

Licheng Kuo, MSc Department of Medical Physics, Memorial Sloan Kettering Cancer Center, New York, NY, USA

Hsiao-Ming Lu, PhD Department of Radiation Oncology, Francis H. Burr Proton Therapy Center, Massachusetts General Hospital, Boston, MA, USA

Shannon M. MacDonald Department of Radiation Oncology, Massachusetts General Hospital, Harvard Medical School, Boston, MA, USA

Carol Marquez, MD Department of Radiation Oncology, Stanford University, Stanford, CA, USA

Robert W. Mutter Department of Radiation Oncology, Mayo Clinic Rochester, Rochester, MN, USA

Sook Kien Ng Department of Radiation Oncology and Molecular Radiation Sciences, Johns Hopkins University, Baltimore, MD, USA

Mark Pankuch, PhD Medical Physics and Dosimetry, Northwestern Medicine Chicago Proton Center, Warrenville, IL, USA

Tracy Sherertz, MD Department of Radiation Oncology, University of California, San Francisco, San Francisco, CA, USA

Jonathan B. Strauss, MD Department of Radiation Oncology, Northwestern University Feinberg School of Medicine, Chicago, IL, USA

An Tai, PhD Department of Radiation Oncology, Medical College of Wisconsin, Milwaukee, WI, USA

Jean Wright Department of Radiation Oncology and Molecular Radiation Sciences, Johns Hopkins University, Baltimore, MD, USA

Sua Yoo, PhD Department of Radiation Oncology, Duke University Medical Center, Durham, NC, USA

Whole Breast Radiation for Early Stage Breast Cancer

Rachel C. Blitzblau, Sua Yoo, and Janet K. Horton

Contents

Many patients with early stage breast cancer will be candidates for breast conservation including adjuvant radiotherapy. In this setting, whole breast radiotherapy (WBRT) is the most commonly utilized approach. This can be accomplished with the patient in the supine or prone position, and the treatment course can range from 3 to 7 weeks in duration, depending on patient and tumor characteristics. Generally, 3–6 weeks elapse following lumpectomy before initiation of WBRT to allow post-surgical healing. In this chapter, we cover the basics of the whole breast radiotherapy treatment planning.

R.C. Blitzblau, MD, PhD • S. Yoo, PhD • J.K. Horton, MD (✉)
Department of Radiation Oncology, Duke University Medical Center, Durham, NC, USA
e-mail: Janet.horton@duke.edu

© Springer International Publishing Switzerland 2016
J.R. Bellon et al. (eds.), *Radiation Therapy Techniques and Treatment Planning for Breast Cancer*, Practical Guides in Radiation Oncology,
DOI 10.1007/978-3-319-40392-2_1

1.1   Initial Simulation

The majority of US treatment centers utilize computed tomography (CT)-based simulation and treatment planning. In the supine position, patients are immobilized with their arms up on a breast board, Alpha Cradle, Vac-Lok, or other immobilization devices (Fig. 1.1a, b). Often, some degree of tilt is applied to isolate breast tissue below the level of the head of the clavicle. The patient's head is positioned with the chin up and may be turned slightly to the contralateral side if necessary to keep it out of the radiation field. In the prone position, the patient is positioned with their arms up and head turned either away from the treated breast, toward the treated breast, or in a neutral position depending on the style of prone breast board and individual patient comfort (Fig. 1.1c, d). The ipsilateral breast falls into the open portion of the breast board, while the contralateral breast is pulled away and supported beneath the patient. Prone positioning may be particularly useful for patients with large breasts in order to reduce the tissue separation size and minimize the inframammary fold.

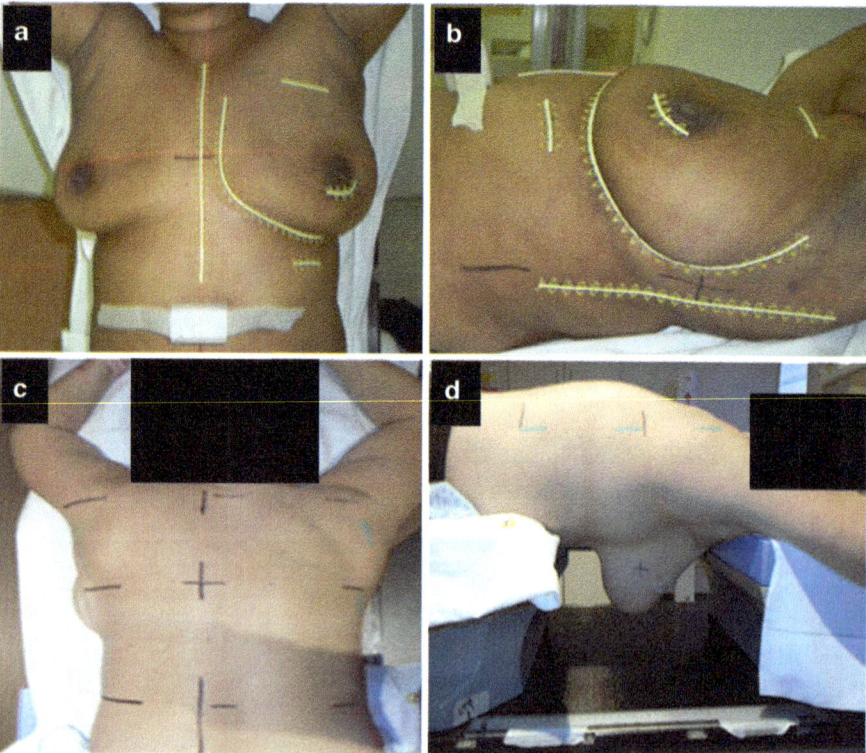

Fig. 1.1 Patient positioning and marking for CT simulation in the supine (**a, b**) or prone (**c, d**) positions. Radiopaque fiducial wires are placed to mark the superior, inferior, medial and lateral extent of breast tissue plus a margin (**a, b**). A wire is utilized over the lumpectomy incision and one delineating the breast tissue from 2 to 10 o'clock (**a, b**). Leveling marks are drawn on the patients torso in the supine (**a, b**) and prone positions (**c, d**) for alignment on the treatment machine

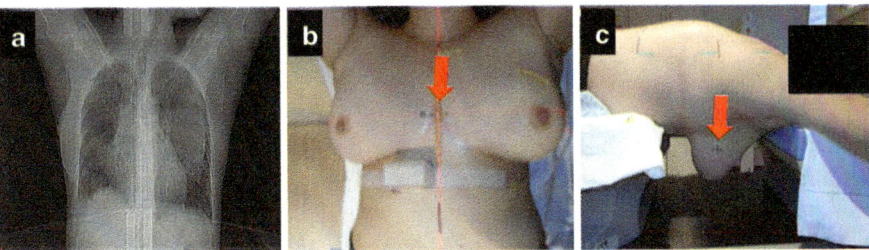

Fig. 1.2 CT scout imaging and reference markings. (**a**) A scout image is taken to confirm the scan area and patient position. (**b**) A stable reference point is set on the central sternum (*arrow*) in the supine position. (**c**) A stable reference point in the prone position is set on the lateral breast (*arrow*)

Prior to the CT scan, radiopaque fiducial wires are placed on the patient in order to delineate the clinical boundaries of the breast tissue (Fig. 1.1). Traditionally, the superior border is placed at the inferior aspect of the clavicular head, the inferior border approximately 2 cm below the inframammary fold, the medial border at midline over the sternum, and the lateral border at the midaxillary line. A fiducial wire is also placed on the lumpectomy scar. Adjustment of the wires from standard physical landmarks may be required to allow approximately 2 cm margin around the palpable breast tissue for patients with larger or smaller breast sizes. Current cooperative group trials often utilize semicircular demarcation of the clinically apparent breast tissue in addition to the landmarks described above. For women simulated in the prone position, all wire demarcation is performed in the supine position with arms up prior to prone immobilization.

Next, a scout CT scan is obtained to verify patient position, alignment, and reproducibility (Fig. 1.2a). Subsequently, 2–4 mm axial CT images are obtained with superior and inferior scan borders several centimeters above and below the desired top and bottom of the treatment fields. If a respiratory gating system is in use, the scan borders should be adjusted to include the necessary apparatus (see chapter on deep inspiratory breath hold for more details).

A stable reference point is then set to facilitate patient positioning on the day of simulation (Fig. 1.2b, c). At our institution, this point is placed along the sternum at mid-chest level in the supine position. For patients treated prone, the reference point is placed in the middle of the breast tissue in the cephalocaudal direction and on the lateral aspect of the breast at the level of the breast board surface in the anteroposterior direction. In either case, the reference point is marked on the patient's skin utilizing the room lasers and subsequently utilized for shifts to the treatment isocenter during positioning on the treatment table. Alternatively, the isocenter may be selected and marked on the patient at the time of CT simulation. Indexing and leveling marks are also made on the patient along the thorax, breast, and arms (prone) and protected with clear stickers to maximize reproducibility on the treatment table. A greater number of markings may be required for prone positioning, due to larger interfraction setup variability [1]. Alternatively, permanent tattoos may be utilized for treatment position markings.

1.2   Boost Simulation

For patients treated in the supine position, the initial simulation scan is often sufficient for boost treatment planning as well (Fig. 1.3a, c, e). However, for patients
initially simulated and treated in the prone position, a repeat simulation is usually
required in the supine or lateral decubitus position to allow optimal access to the
tumor bed. In addition, for patients initially treated in the supine position with lateral or deep tumor beds and/or very large breasts, decubitus positioning may also be
a consideration (Fig. 1.3b, d, f). A fiducial wire is again placed to identify the
lumpectomy scar and the patient positioned comfortably, though any immobilization in this position is difficult. A tumor bed boost can also be performed in the
prone position but is more technically challenging due to physical linear accelerator
limitations and the conformation of the tumor bed in this position. Occasionally, for
patients with a large seroma at the initiation of treatment, a subsequent scan closer
to initiation of the boost may generate a smaller target volume as the seroma will
often regress with time. In addition, some institutions use compression devices to
flatten the overlying breast tissue as an adjunct or alternative to changes in the treatment position.

1.3   Tangent Field Design

CT images are imported to the treatment planning system. The first step is contouring of normal structures, which for WBRT generally includes body, heart, lungs,
and potentially contralateral breast or brachial plexus depending on the clinical situation (Fig. 1.4). Target structures for WBRT include the entire ipsilateral breast, the
tumor bed, and level 1/2 axillary nodes (in certain clinical scenarios) plus expansions for margin. Please see the chapter on target delineation and anatomy for further details of this process.

The treatment isocenter is commonly set midway between the superior and inferior as well as medial and lateral aspects of the field (Fig. 1.5a, b) in supine position.
Many centers set the isocenter depth just posterior to the chest wall to ensure adequate coverage of the breast but allow half-beam blocking at the posterior edge.
Alternatively, the isocenter may be set in the breast tissue and the gantry angle
rotated to match the posterior beam edge divergence. In the prone position, isocenter selection is more challenging. A point must be chosen that is reproducible and
feasible for imaging and will not result in treatment collision. At our institution, this
point is at the center in the axial view, which is usually medial to the breast tissue
and anterior to the chest wall, and outside the patient (Fig. 1.5c, d).

Standard fields consist of medial and lateral tangential beams designed to encompass the entire ipsilateral breast (Fig. 1.6). Attention is given to adequate coverage
of the tumor bed and clearance of the breast tissue. Treatment of axillary levels
1/2 in addition to the whole breast can be achieved by raising the upper border of the
fields, also known as high tangents (Fig. 1.6), and utilizing multi-leaf collimators
(MLCs) to shape the field. This is best accomplished by contouring the desired
nodal levels to ensure that the field length and shape is adequate versus relying on a
specific measurement or bony landmark.

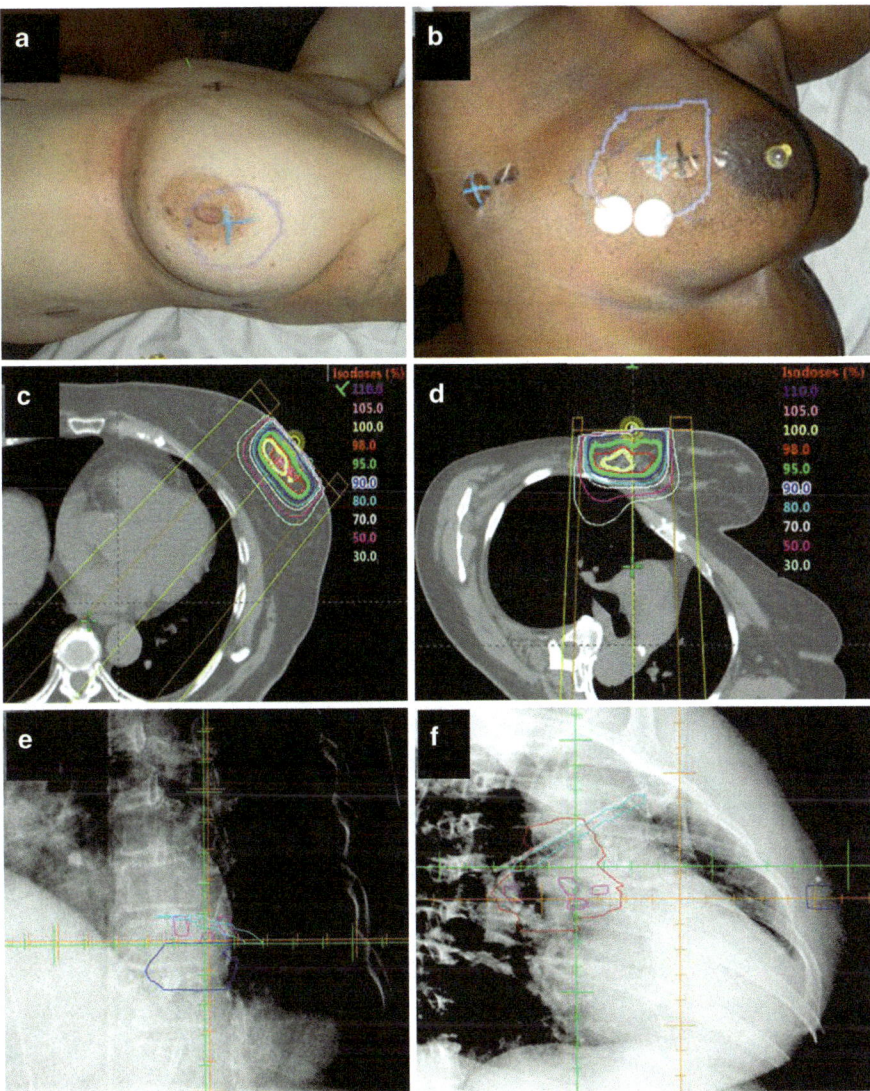

Fig. 1.3 Tumor bed boost performed in the supine (**a**, **c**, **e**) or decubitus (**b**, **d**, **f**) position. Skin marking of the tumor bed boost field shape for a supine (**a**) or decubitus patient (**b**). Axial dose distribution from an en face electron field for a supine (**c**) or decubitus (**d**) patient. In the decubitus position, there is flattening of the lateral breast and enhanced electron dosimetry. (**e**) A typical small shift to match clips using KV imaging for a supine boost patient. (**e**) A larger shift on KV clip match for a decubitus boost patient demonstrating the lesser stability of this position and highlighting the need for daily imaging to ensure appropriate positioning. The scar (*aqua*) and nipple (*blue*) are also marked to aid in positioning

Gantry angle, collimator angle, and table angle can all be adjusted to optimize coverage of desired targets while minimizing normal tissue inclusion within the fields. Custom MLCs can shape the field further and may be particularly useful for blocking the heart (Fig. 1.7a, b). The medial and lateral fields are matched to each

Fig. 1.4 Axial CT image illustrating treatment targets and normal tissue contours. *Pink* heart, *purple* lungs, *green* contralateral breast, *yellow* ipsilateral breast, *red* tumor bed

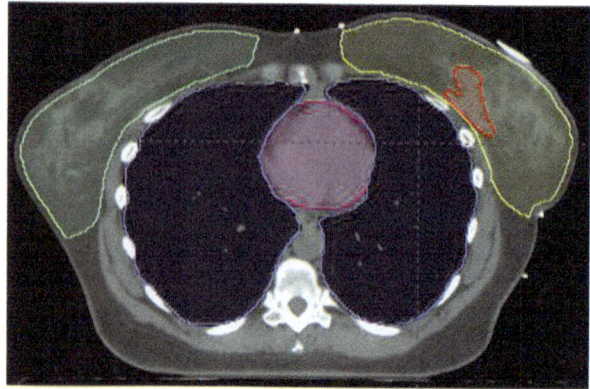

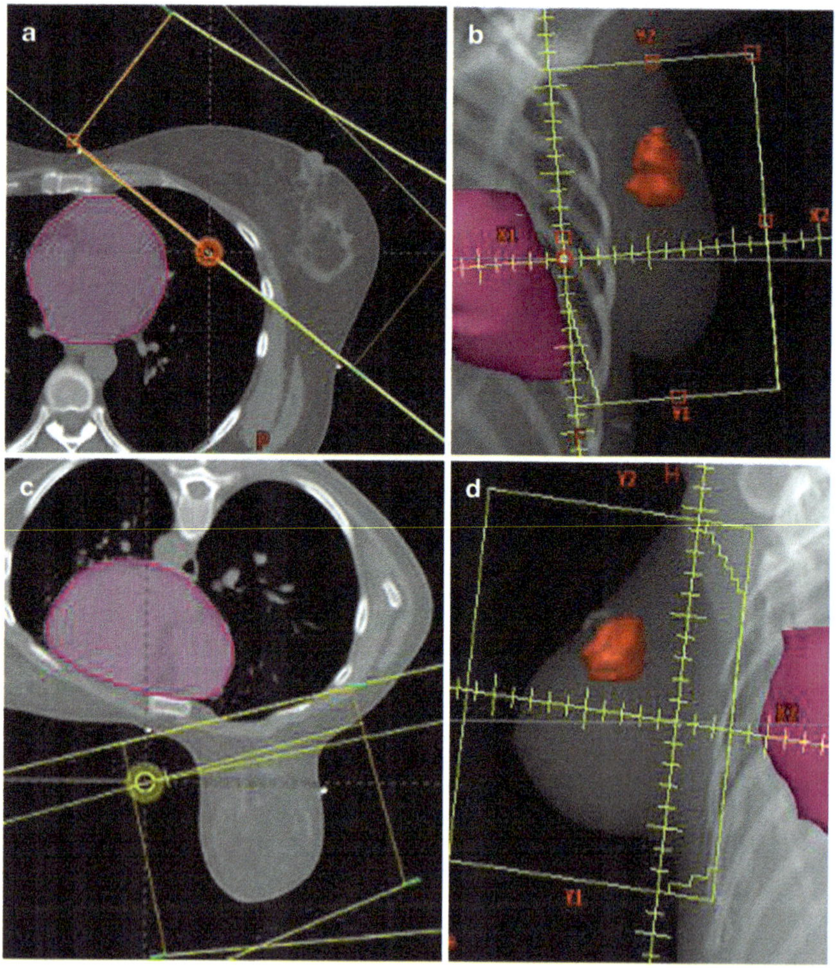

Fig. 1.5 Isocenter placement for tangent fields. (**a**) Axial CT images and (**b**) beam's eye view of isocenter (*circle*, center of graticule) placement for a supine patient. (**c**) Axial and (**d**) beam's eye view of isocenter (*circle*, center of graticule) placement for a prone patient. Due to the superior displacement of the patient on the prone breast board, the isocenter is placed in air medial to the breast tissue in order to avoid collision

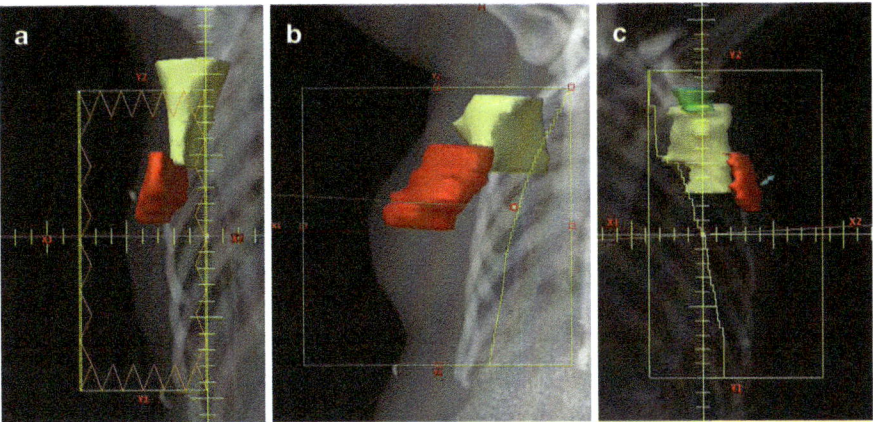

Fig. 1.6 Tangent field design. (**a**) A standard tangent without purposeful axillary coverage shows only incidental coverage of the axilla. (**b**) A high tangent designed for coverage of axillary level I alone. (**c**) A high tangent shaped for coverage of axillary levels I/II

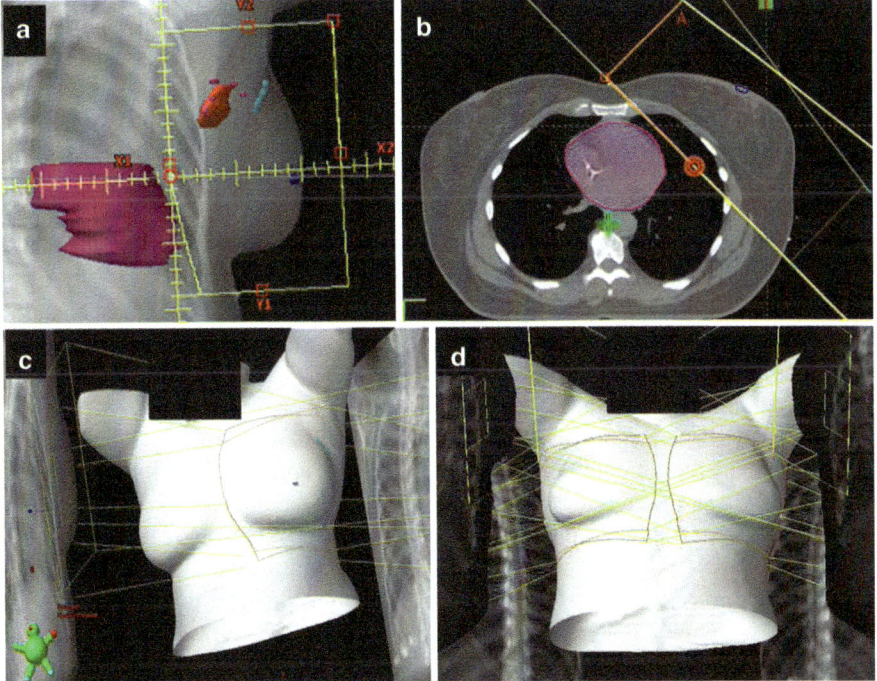

Fig. 1.7 Tangent field optimization with normal tissue protection. (**a**) Beam's eye and (**b**) axial CT images illustrating a custom MLC heart block and non-divergent posterior field edges. (**c**) Skin rendering demonstrating non-divergence of the medial tangent beam entrance and lateral tangent beam exit, including the heart block. (**d**) Skin rendering demonstrating the gap between tangent fields for bilateral breast treatment with non-divergence of medial tangent beam entrance and lateral tangent beam exit as in panel **c**

other in height and shape with offset to prevent beam divergence along the posterior field border. It often is simplest to fully optimize the medial beam shape and then match the lateral beam. Care is taken to align the exit of the lateral beam with the entrance of the medial beam to minimize dose to the opposite breast (Fig. 1.7c). Medial alignment is of particular importance in the relatively uncommon situation in which bilateral WBRT treatment is desired. Field design in this setting is as described above, with care to allow a small gap at the central chest between the two sets of fields such that daily overlap is unlikely (Fig. 1.7d). Modern treatment planning software facilitates this with settings that allow you to see beam entry and/or exit shape on the body contour and in the beam's eye view.

1.4 Boost Field Design

The most commonly utilized method for treatment of the tumor bed is an en face electron field (Fig. 1.3). The treatment isocenter is set at the skin surface and the electron cutout designed to encompass the expanded tumor bed volume with a margin. More or less margin may be required to accommodate immobilization position, setup stability, and patient and tumor characteristics. Gantry, table, and collimator angles are selected to allow a maximally en face approach. For very deep or lateral tumor beds, mini-tangent fields or a 4–5 photon field bouquet may be required.

1.5 Dose Calculation and Modulation

Once treatment fields are set, dose calculation is performed. Due to the shape of the breast, there can be large variability in tissue thickness. This leads to inhomogeneous dose distribution, particularly in the setting of larger breast sizes and/or wide separations. The presence of low density lung tissue just behind the breast can also lead to challenges in maintaining adequate coverage near the chest wall. However, multiple methods exist to improve dose homogeneity and are routinely applied in WBRT planning.

Physical wedges are one method traditionally utilized to improve homogeneity (Fig. 1.8a). The placement of the wedge with the heel compensating for the thinnest area of the breast tissue reduces the hot spots in that region. However, field size is limited with a maximum dimension that depends on the wedge angle. Modern linear accelerators allow the use of dynamic wedges, which utilize collimator jaw movement while the beam is on to modulate dose. Dynamic wedging permits larger field sizes, does not require manual placement of heavy wedges by the treating therapists, and reduces electron contamination. Patient-customized physical compensators can also be used, though these may be too labor-intensive to be of practical use in many treatment centers.

One of the simplest and most widely available ways to improve dose homogeneity is combining higher and lower energy photon beams. For additional refinement of the treatment plan, a "field-in-field" technique is often utilized (Fig. 1.8b–e).

Following initial dose calculation, a few subfields are created from each tangential beam with MLCs blocking the high dose (e.g., 110 and 105 % dose) regions. A small proportion of the overall dose is then delivered through these fields, improving dose homogeneity.

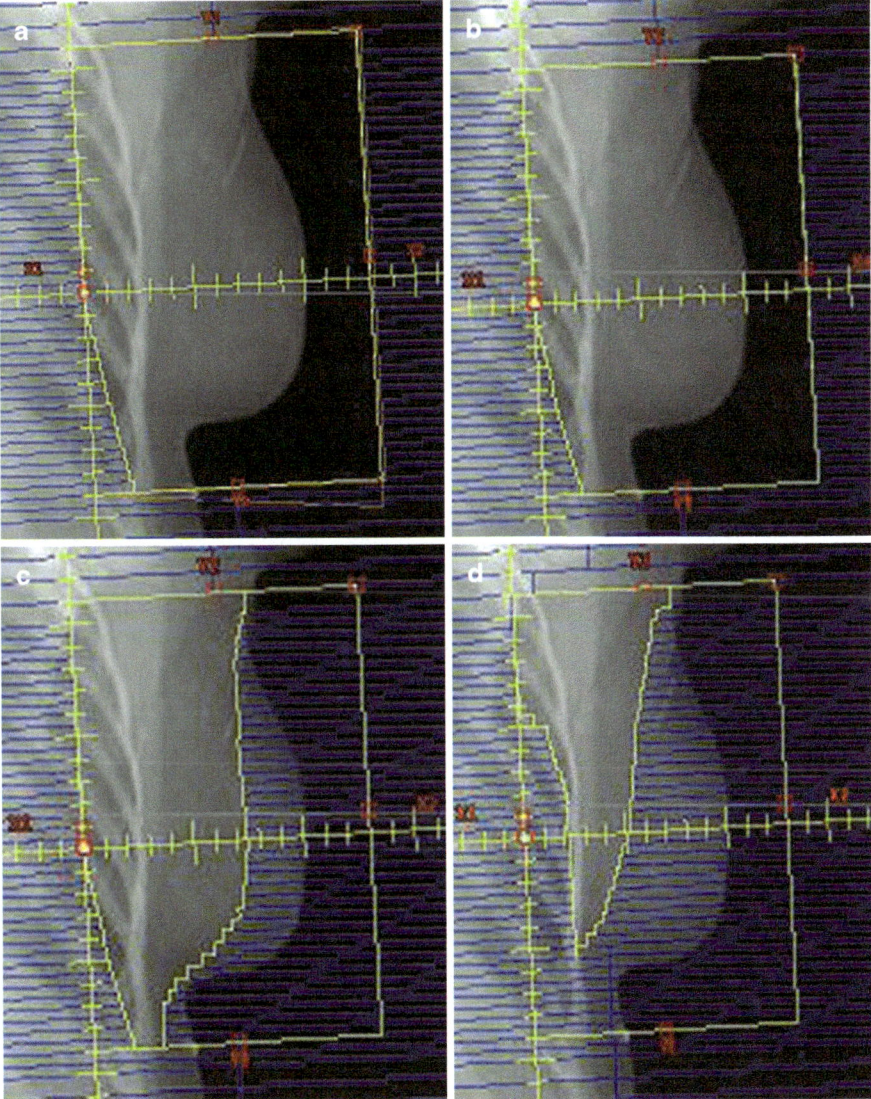

Fig. 1.8 Optimization of dose homogeneity. (**a**) A beam's eye view of a tangent field containing a physical wedge with its heel toward the narrow anterior breast (*orange triangle*). (**b-e**) Beam's eye views of an open tangent with several smaller subfields as utilized for field-in-field treatment. (**f**) A beam's eye view of a tangent field fluence map as utilized for ECOMP

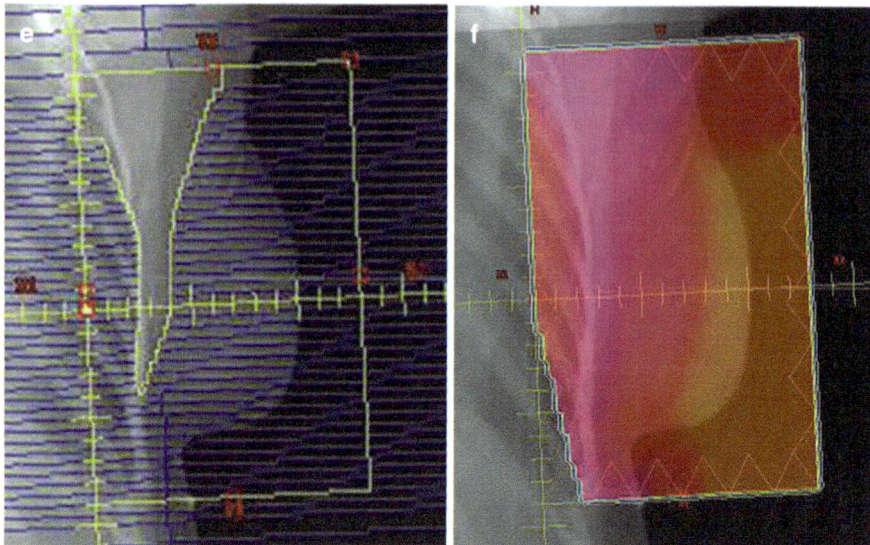

Fig. 1.8 (continued)

Finally, electronic tissue compensation (ECOMP) is a forward planned dose painting method which involves manual modification of fluence distribution within each tangent field to achieve maximal dose homogeneity (Fig. 1.8f). The treatment planning software subsequently converts the fluence maps to MLC sequences for treatment delivery. ECOMP generally requires less planning time and utilizes fewer monitor units for dose delivery while preserving target coverage and normal tissue sparing as compared to inverse planned intensity-modulated radiotherapy (IMRT) [2, 3]. Routine usage of IMRT for WBRT was recommended against in the 2013 Choosing Wisely campaign [4] and should be limited to specific cases where other methods are inadequate.

1.6   Tumor Bed Boost

Electron energy is selected based on desired depth of coverage as determined by the tumor bed target volumes within the breast. The normalization point is set at nominal Dmax for the chosen electron energy, with the dose often prescribed to the 100 % isodose line. An alternate isodose line (or prescription depth) can be selected if a greater dose at depth is desired. However, it is important to keep in mind that the maximum dose also increases with this approach. A boost plan can be done with mini-tangent or 4–5 beam bouquet fields with energy photon or mixed photon electron fields, as needed, to optimize conformality of the dose coverage while sparing surrounding normal tissues.

1.7   Plan Evaluation

The treating physician reviews the CT-based treatment plan on a slice-by-slice basis within the treatment planning software. In addition, three-dimensional treatment planning allows generation of dose-volume histograms for review of dose delivered to contoured target structures and normal tissues (Fig. 1.9). Individual physicians will vary in what they consider an acceptable plan, and this will likely also vary depending on individual patient tumor and body characteristics, as well as individual recurrence risk. Currently open cooperative group trials are one resource for desired plan parameters and commonly use a coverage parameter of ≥95 % of the ipsilateral breast target volume receiving ≥95 % of the prescribed dose [5, 6]. Another commonly used parameter is that all clinically delineated breast tissue is covered by the 98 % dose line. Ninety to ninety-five percent coverage is often acceptable for nodal targets. Again, however, what is deemed acceptable coverage may vary depending on the individual patient clinical scenario.

Dose homogeneity, in terms of overall point dose maximum, as well as volume receiving 105 and 110 % of the prescribed dose, is also an important component of thorough plan evaluation. Dose homogeneity is often excellent but is significantly impacted by patient factors, particularly separation size. In patients with large separations, there may still be significant 105 and 110 % dose regions even with modern

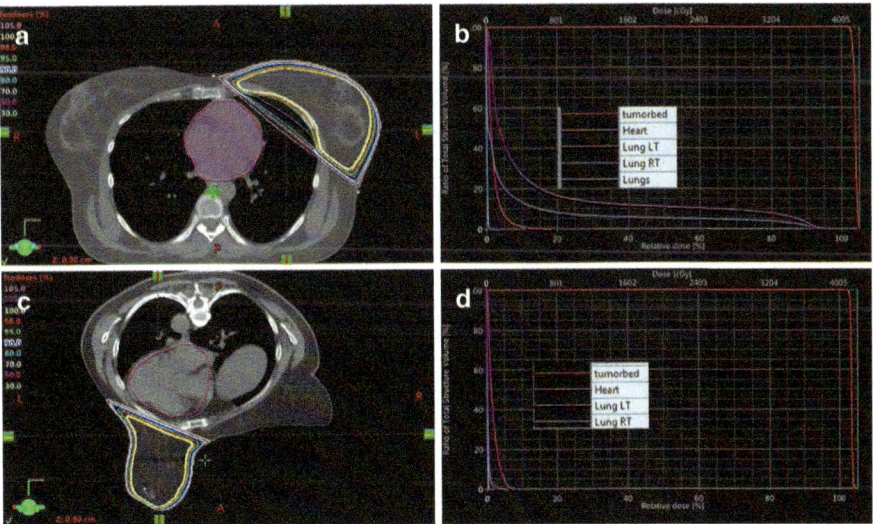

Fig. 1.9   Plan evaluation. (**a**) Axial CT image demonstrating dose coverage of the breast for a supine patient. (**b**) DVH showing tumor bed coverage as well as heart and lung doses for the same supine patient. (**c**) Axial CT image demonstrating dose coverage of the breast for a prone patient. (**d**) DVH showing tumor bed coverage as well as heart and lung doses for the same prone patient. Note the significantly lower lung dose in the prone position and low heart dose in both positions

techniques. Current NRG protocols are an excellent resource to aid in determining if the extent of the breast receiving greater than prescription dose is reasonable [6].

Finally, during plan evaluation normal tissue protection is reviewed. The most important normal tissues to consider with WBRT are the contralateral breast, lungs, and heart, particularly when treating the left breast. There are no strictly agreed upon dose constraints for the lung; however, there are data that indicate that symptomatic pneumonitis is rare with ipsilateral lung V20 less than 30%, and this is usually easily achievable with breast only radiotherapy [7, 8]. Recent NRG protocols require a V20≤20% and a V5≤55% for patients not receiving regional nodal radiation [6]. Mean cardiac dose should be as low as reasonably possible, generally ≤4 Gy, but doses far less than this are typically achievable. The contralateral breast should be kept out of the direct beam path.

1.8 Dose and Fractionation

Standard WBRT consists of 45–50 Gy in 25–28 fractions of 1.8–2 Gy. Long-term data from multiple large randomized trials also demonstrate the non-inferiority of hypofractionated WBRT (HF-WBRT) consisting of 40.05–42.56 Gy in 15–16 fractions of 2.66–2.67 Gy for early stage breast cancer with equal or lesser acute and long-term toxicity [9, 10]. These trials contained separation size and dose homogeneity requirements that were generally simpler than those currently used with modern treatment planning techniques. There are no strictly agreed upon dose homogeneity criterion for utilization of HF-WBRT, and it is likely that wide variation in clinical application exists.

Tumor bed boost dose ranges from 10 to 16 Gy in 4–8 fractions of 2–2.5 Gy. Tumor bed dose greater than 60 Gy may be desired in patients with positive margins or other high-risk features. However, there are no strictly agreed upon boost dose guidelines at this time, particularly in the setting of HF-WBRT.

1.9 Treatment Imaging

During the course of whole breast radiotherapy treatment delivery port films are utilized to evaluate setup accuracy (Fig. 1.10). Digitally reconstructed radiographs (DRRs) are generated with the CT data set and used for anterior to posterior (AP) or posterior to anterior (PA) and lateral orthogonal setup films. A beam's eye view is also generated for each tangential treatment field. MV port films and KV on-board imaging are approved by the treating physician prior to delivering the first treatment to confirm isocenter location, patient positioning, and field shape. Subsequent imaging frequency throughout the treatment course depends on treating physician preference and factors including ease of treatment field visualization, individual patient setup variability, immobilization technique, and utilization of respiratory gating or breath-hold techniques. Free breathing supine position treatments generally require the least frequent imaging, with prone breast or breath-hold treatments requiring more frequent portal images.

Imaging for the boost typically involves a KV image in the treatment position to confirm isocenter position (Fig. 1.3e). Once the isocenter is confirmed, MLCs are used to illustrate the planned treatment volume on the patient and thus confirm appropriate shape and placement of the electron cutout. In the decubitus position, daily KV imaging is required due to the challenges of immobilization in this position and subsequent potential for large daily shifts (Fig. 1.3f).

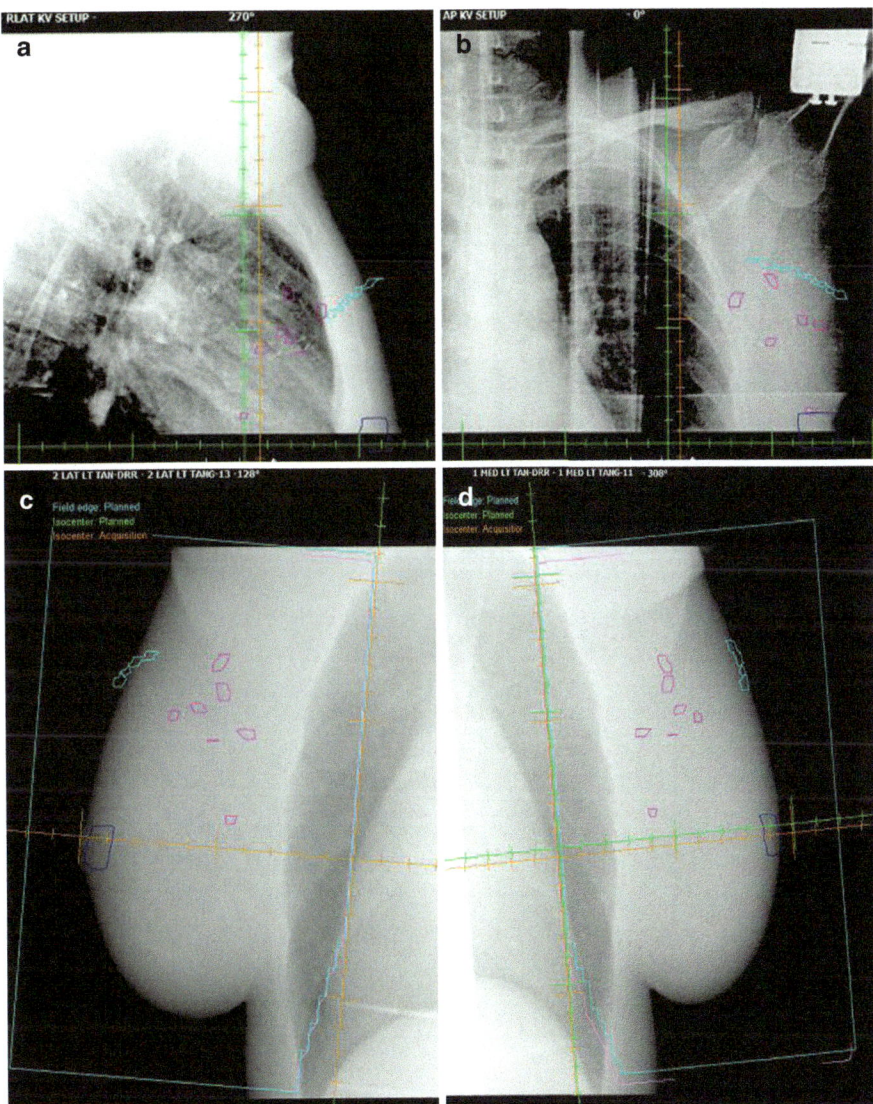

Fig. 1.10 Treatment imaging. (**a**) Lateral and (**b**) AP KV orthogonal setup images for a supine patient as well as (**c**) medial and (**d**) lateral MV port films. (**e**) Lateral and (**f**) AP KV orthogonal setup images for a prone patient with a (**g**) KV lateral tangent beams eye view port film for visualization of the chest wall and (**h**) medial and (**i**) lateral MV port films for visualization of the breast tissue

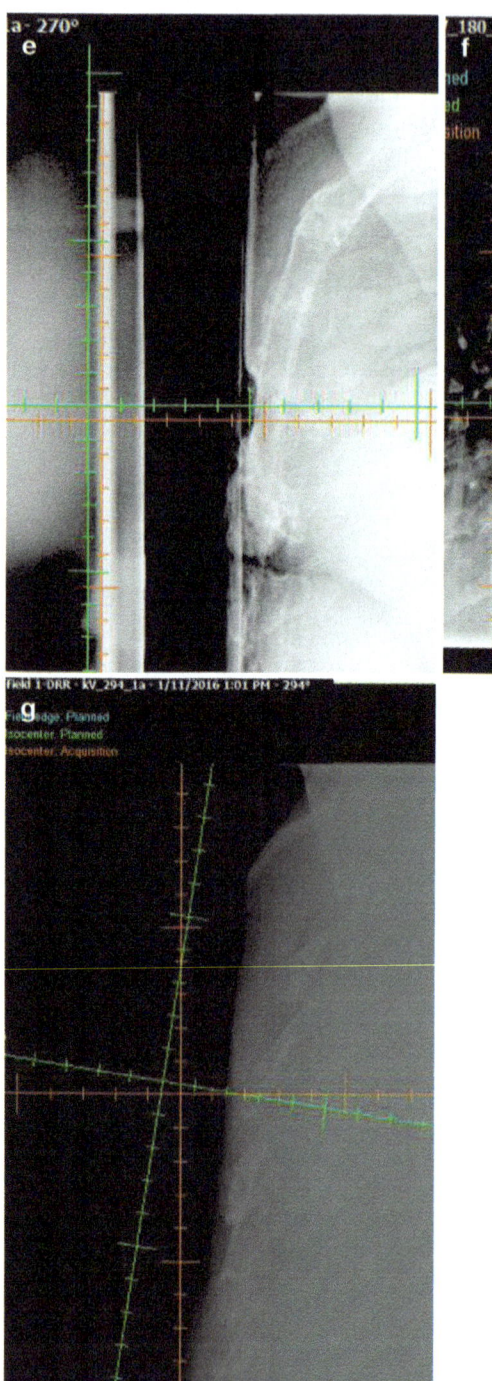

Fig. 1.10 (continued)

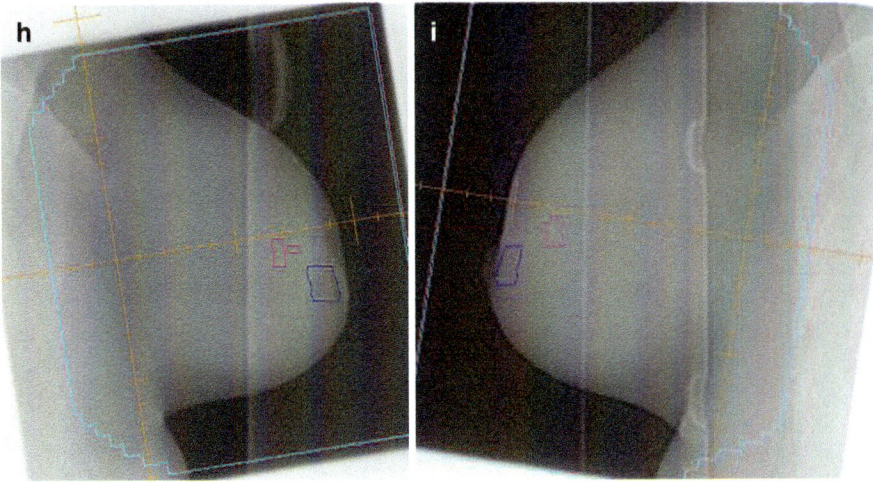

Fig. 1.10   (continued)

References

1. Mitchell J, Formenti SC, Dewyngaert JK (2010) Interfraction and intrafraction setup variability for prone breast radiation therapy. Int J Radiat Oncol Biol Phys 76(5):1571–1577
2. Caudell JJ et al (2007) A dosimetric comparison of electronic compensation, conventional intensity modulated radiotherapy, and tomotherapy in patients with early-stage carcinoma of the left breast. Int J Radiat Oncol Biol Phys 68(5):1505–1511
3. Al-Rahbi ZS et al (2013) Dosimetric comparison of intensity modulated radiotherapy isocentric field plans and field in field (FIF) forward plans in the treatment of breast cancer. J Med Phys 38(1):22–29
4. Hahn C et al (2014) Choosing wisely: the American Society for Radiation Oncology's top 5 list. Pract Radiat Oncol 4(6):349–355
5. www.Rtog.Org
6. www.Nrgoncology.Org
7. Lind PA et al (2001) Pulmonary complications following different radiotherapy techniques for breast cancer, and the association to irradiated lung volume and dose. Breast Cancer Res Treat 68(3):199–210
8. Blom Goldman U et al (2010) Reduction of radiation pneumonitis by V20-constraints in breast cancer. Radiat Oncol 5:99
9. Whelan TJ et al (2010) Long-term results of hypofractionated radiation therapy for breast cancer. N Engl J Med 362(6):513–520
10. Haviland JS et al (2013) The Uk standardisation of breast radiotherapy (START) trials of radiotherapy hypofractionation for treatment of early breast cancer: 10-year follow-up results of two randomised controlled trials. Lancet Oncol 14(11):1086–1094

Postmastectomy Radiotherapy with and Without Reconstruction

2

Kathleen C. Horst, Nataliya Kovalchuk, and Carol Marquez

Contents

2.1 Current Indications for Postmastectomy Radiotherapy

The role of radiotherapy after mastectomy, postmastectomy radiotherapy (PMRT), in women with node-positive or high-risk node-negative breast cancer has evolved over the last several decades since the publication of the randomized trials from the British Columbia Cancer Agency and the Danish Breast Cancer Cooperative Group [1–3]. These trials were the first trials using modern radiation techniques and systemic therapy to demonstrate that PMRT not only reduced locoregional recurrences (LRRs) but also improved survival. The impact of PMRT on local control and overall survival has been further supported by the results of the Early Breast Cancer Trialists' Collaborative Group (EBCTCG) meta-analysis [4, 5].

K.C. Horst, MD (✉)
Department of Radiation Oncology, Stanford University School of Medicine, Stanford, CA, USA
e-mail: kateh@stanford.edu

N. Kovalchuk, PhD • C. Marquez, MD
Department of Radiation Oncology, Stanford University, Stanford, CA, USA

© Springer International Publishing Switzerland 2016
J.R. Bellon et al. (eds.), *Radiation Therapy Techniques and Treatment Planning for Breast Cancer*, Practical Guides in Radiation Oncology,
DOI 10.1007/978-3-319-40392-2_2

After the initial publication of the Danish and Canadian studies, the benefit of PMRT was readily accepted for women at high risk of LRR. National guidelines were developed to endorse the routine use of PMRT for patients with four or more involved lymph nodes or those with T3/T4 tumors with any nodal involvement [6, 7].

While there had been some uncertainty about the role of PMRT in patients with 1–3 involved nodes, the recent update of the EBCTCG meta-analysis demonstrated a reduction in recurrence and breast cancer mortality after PMRT even in this intermediate-risk population. Furthermore, the MA.20 National Cancer Institute of Canada and EORTC 22922/10925 trials demonstrated an improvement in disease-free survival and distant metastasis-free survival with the addition of regional nodal irradiation in any node-positive or high-risk node-negative patient [8, 9]. Although these trials primarily included patients treated with breast conservation, the results suggest that regional nodal irradiation may have a substantial impact on distant breast cancer outcomes. Additional prospective data evaluating the role of PMRT in intermediate-risk patients is expected from a study in the UK (Selective Use of Postoperative Radiotherapy after Mastectomy) [10].

Nonetheless, the results from the Danish and Canadian studies as well as the EBCTCG meta-analysis are not uniformly adopted in the modern era since improved chemotherapy, use of targeted biologics, and extended endocrine therapy contribute to lower rates of LRR than what was reported in those older studies. Further more, the risk of LRR, as well as benefit from PMRT, varies according to biologic subtype [11, 12]. In addition to the T stage and the nodal status, the use of systemic therapy and the biologic subtype may also be important factors to consider when determining LRR risk and the role of PMRT.

There are currently no prospective randomized data assessing the role of PMRT after neoadjuvant chemotherapy. Retrospective studies suggest that those who present with clinical stage III disease or those with residual nodal disease after chemotherapy are at high enough risk of LRR to warrant PMRT [13–15]. In a retrospective analysis of NSABP B-18 and B-27, patients with clinical stage II disease who achieved a pathologic complete response (pCR) after neoadjuvant chemotherapy had a low risk of LRR after mastectomy without radiotherapy [16]. Given this low risk, the benefit of PMRT after neoadjuvant chemotherapy remains an area of uncertainty [17]. The ongoing NSABP B-51/RTOG 1304 (NRG 9353) trial is randomizing patients with biopsy-proven nodal involvement who achieve a pCR in the nodes after neoadjuvant chemotherapy to observation or PMRT [18]. The results of this trial will help guide PMRT treatment recommendations in patients who receive neoadjuvant chemotherapy.

2.2   Simulation

For patients receiving PMRT, the use of a CT simulator and three-dimensional treatment planning is preferable in order to allow visualization of the target and normal tissues.

Patients should be immobilized using a breast board or a customized foam mold or vacuum cushion. Patients are placed in the supine position with the ipsilateral or bilateral arms abducted approximately 90–120° with the shoulder externally rotated. The patient's head could be turned to the contralateral side to minimize any skin-folds that may increase the skin reaction in that region. The clinical borders of the chest wall should be marked with radiopaque wire to establish field borders that can be visualized on the CT images. These borders are typically at the inferior aspect of the clavicular head (superior border), midaxillary line (lateral border), midsternum (medial border), and 1 cm inferior to the inframammary fold of the contralateral breast or 1 cm inferior to the reconstructed breast (inferior border). In addition to the radiopaque wire placed to delineate field borders, a wire should be placed on the mastectomy scar, drain sites, and any other scars that need to be included in the treatment fields. Intravenous contrast is not routinely used; however, if there is a patient with enlarged nodes suspicious for gross involvement, IV contrast may help for nodal delineation for boost treatment. In patients with gross nodal disease at presentation who respond to systemic therapy, fusion with a diagnostic CT or PET may also aid in nodal delineation.

Axial CT images are then acquired using 2–3 mm slices to provide three-dimensional images of the chest wall and nodal regions. These images should extend from the mid-cervical spine to below the inferior border. Respiratory gating or deep inspiration breath hold should be considered for patients with left-sided tumors. These techniques are discussed in a separate chapter.

2.3   Treatment Volumes

Based on patterns of locoregional recurrence after mastectomy, treatment volumes for PMRT generally include the entire chest wall and mastectomy scar, as well as the at-risk regional nodes (supraclavicular, infraclavicular, axillary, and internal mammary (IM) nodes). Indications and techniques for treatment of the IM nodes are addressed in another chapter. Contouring atlases have been developed for the delineation of target volumes and normal structures [19, 20]. In particular, the heart should be delineated in patients with left-sided tumors.

2.4   Techniques

Several techniques have been described to treat the chest wall and regional nodes after mastectomy, including tangential photon beams or en face electrons [21]. With each technique, it is important to pay attention to matching fields in order to avoid divergence of one field into the other and overlap of dose.

With photons, one approach is to use a single isocenter for both the chest wall fields and the supraclavicular field (SCF) (monoisocentric technique) (Figs. 2.1 and 2.2). With this approach, the isocenter is placed at the junction between the two fields, which may vary depending on the patient's anatomy, but is usually at the

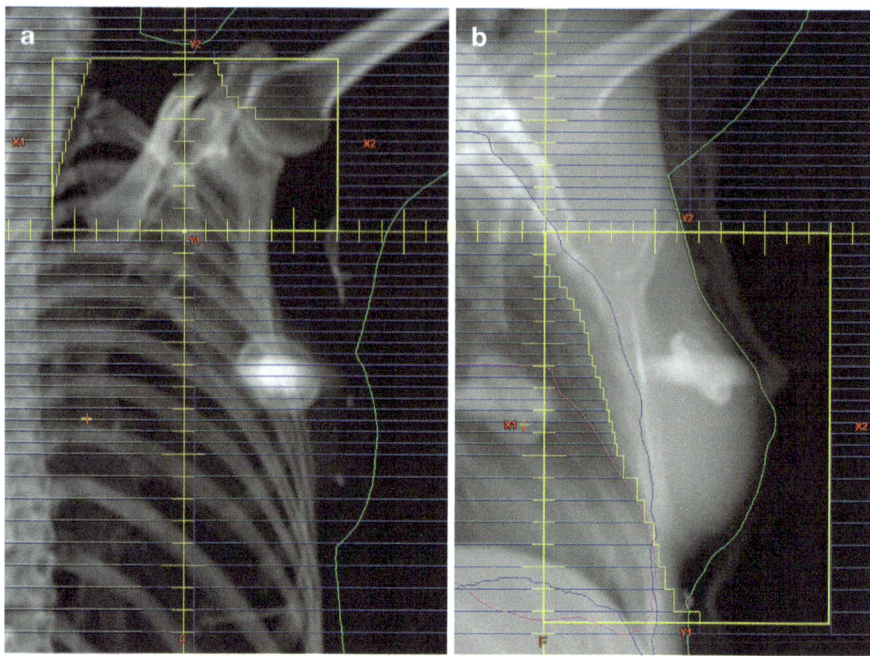

Fig. 2.1 Monoisocentric technique: Beam's eye view (BEV) of the supraclavicular field half-beam blocked at the inferior border (**a**). BEV of the medial tangential quarter-field half-beam blocked at the superior border and posterior border defined by MLC (**b**). *Dark blue* contour projects the ipsilateral lung, and magenta contour projects the heart

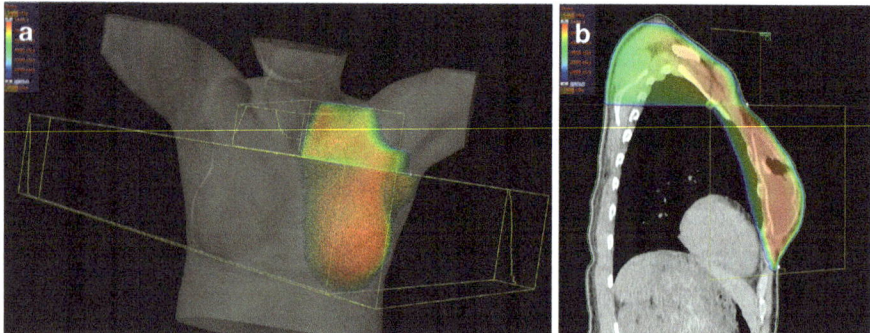

Fig. 2.2 Monoisocentric technique: Skin rendering and dose cloud of the patient treated with the single isocenter placed at the matchline (**a**). Sagittal image of quarter-field tangents and half-beam blocked supraclavicular fields sharing a common isocenter (**b**)

inferior edge of the clavicular head (superior wire). The chest wall is treated with tangential fields, with the superior jaw set to zero to half-beam block/beam split in order to avoid divergence into the SCF. The inferior jaw is opened to the inferior wire. The field size for the tangential field is limited to 20 cm so the placement of

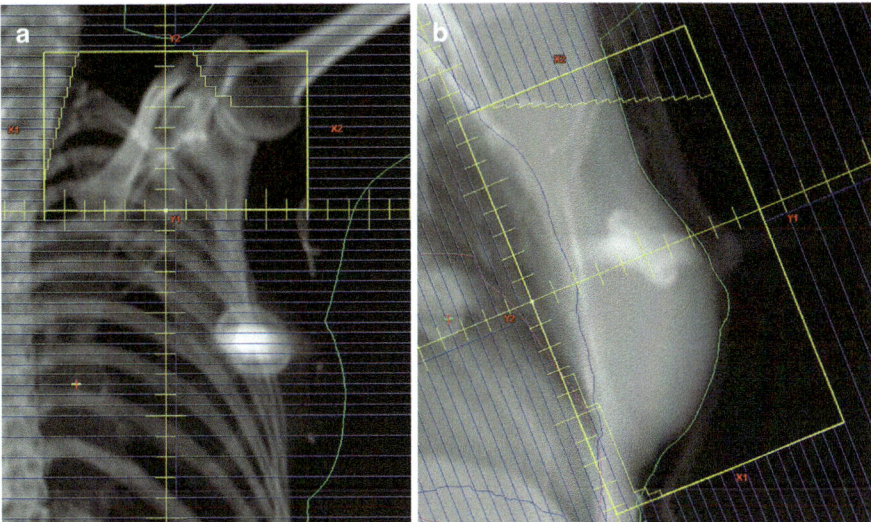

Fig. 2.3 Dual isocentric technique: Supraclavicular field is designed in a similar fashion to monoisocentric technique (**a**). Isocenter for the tangential fields is placed in the lung midway between superior and inferior breast borders, and non-divergent posterior border is achieved by half-beam blocking tangential fields (**b**)

the junction may need to be modified (moved inferiorly) if the field size is greater than 20 cm. No couch rotation is necessary for the tangential field with this technique because the superior edge of the field is not diverging into the SCF. Multileaf collimators (MLCs) can be used to block posteriorly to minimize dose to the lung and heart. For the SCF, an anterior oblique field is matched to the chest wall fields, with the inferior border of the SCF aligning with the superior border of the tangential fields. The inferior jaw is set to zero to half-beam block/beam split in order to avoid divergence into the tangential fields. One advantage of this technique is that with a single isocenter and the elimination of table angles, all fields can be treated in succession without moving the patient.

Another technique utilizes two isocenters: one for the chest wall and one for the SCF (dual isocentric technique) (Figs. 2.3 and 2.4). With this technique, the isocenter for the chest wall is placed in the lung, midway between the superior and inferior borders as defined clinically. The posterior jaw is set at zero to half-beam block/beam split to minimize dose to the lung and heart. The collimator is rotated to align the posterior jaw to the chest wall (Fig. 2.3). This eliminates the need to add additional MLCs to block the lung and heart. With a collimator rotation, a triangular portion of the top of the tangential field juts into the inferior aspect of the supraclavicular field and must be blocked. In addition, in order to avoid divergence from the tangential fields into the SCF, a combination of couch rotations in which the feet move away from the gantry for each tangential field is used to achieve an exact geometric match to the inferior edge of the SCF (Fig. 2.4). Similar to the monoisocentric approach, the isocenter for the SCF is placed at the inferior edge of the

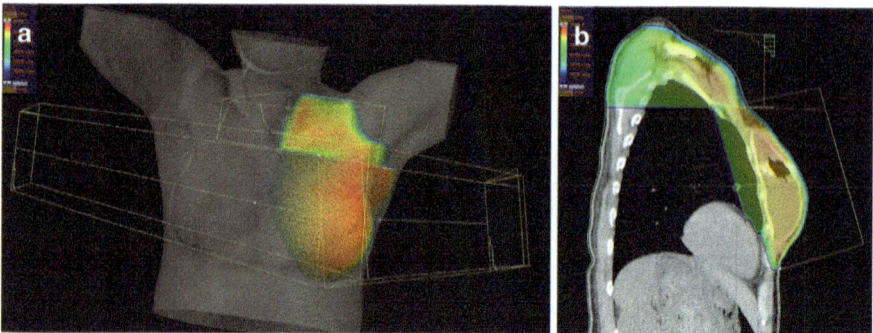

Fig. 2.4 Dual isocentric technique: Skin rendering and dose cloud for the patient treated with two isocenters (tangent isocenter placed in the lung midway between superior and inferior breast borders and supraclavicular isocenter placed at the matchline) (**a**). Sagittal image of dual isocentric setup with the tangents collimated to spare the lung and heart (**b**). The field match is achieved by half-beam blocking the inferior border of supraclavicular field, couch rotations, and MLC blocking of the tangential fields at the superior border

clavicular head (superior wire). The inferior jaw is set to zero to avoid divergence into the tangential fields. This technique utilizing two isocenters eliminates the 20 cm field size limitation; however, it does require shifting the patient, which can potentially introduce errors in the setup.

The chest wall can also be treated using en face electrons; however, there can be dose heterogeneity depending on the contour of the chest wall and the patient's anatomy, particularly for those with reconstruction.

The medial, superior, and lateral jaws of the SCF are set to encompass the at-risk nodes. Generally this leads to the superior jaw being set at the level of the cricoid cartilage, the medial border at the pedicles of the vertebral bodies, and the lateral border at the coracoid process or mid-humeral head (depending on the extent of nodal coverage), with the inferior border set at the superior edge of the tangential fields. Although historically the SCF would flash over the shoulder, with 3D treatment planning, it is best to modify the fields to treat only the nodal areas. Thus, MLCs can be used to block the superior soft tissues as well as the humeral head (Fig. 2.1a). The gantry is rotated to the contralateral side 10–20° to avoid irradiation of the trachea, esophagus, and spinal cord. Historically, the SCF has been prescribed to 3 cm depth; however, with the use of CT treatment planning, it is clear that the depth of the supraclavicular and level III nodes depends on the patient's anatomy. Determining the depth of the nodes is important since it will influence the choice of photon energy or whether a posterior-anterior field may be needed to adequately cover the nodes.

For the photon techniques, there are several ways of improving dose homogeneity for the tangential fields. Intensity-modulated radiotherapy (IMRT) can be used in cases of retreatment or complex geometry. IMRT may offer better target conformality; however, there is often higher integral dose to the lungs and heart. It is unclear whether this increased low-dose exposure will manifest as clinically relevant late effects to these organs [22, 23]. In most PMRT cases, however,

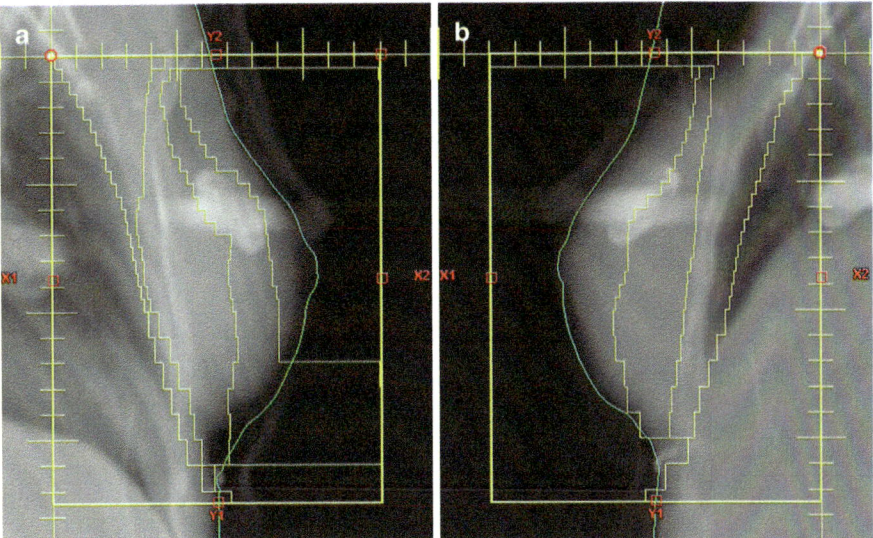

Fig. 2.5 Field-in-Field technique to improve target coverage and dose homogeneity: MLC sub-fields are created based on the open medial and lateral tangential fields to block hot spots in 3–5 % dose increments

three-dimensional conformal radiotherapy techniques can be utilized to achieve dose homogeneity and minimize dose to normal tissue. Using wedges or field-in-field techniques with multileaf collimation and forward planning can achieve these goals (Fig. 2.5). Enhanced dynamic wedges (EDWs) can also be applied to improve dose homogeneity. When the patient separation is large, higher energy photons may be necessary to reduce hot spots.

The use of bolus is generally recommended to ensure that the dose to the skin is adequate. The best schedule is not known, but often 0.5 or 1 cm bolus can be used to increase dose to the superficial tissues.

Techniques for treating the IM nodes are discussed in a separate chapter.

2.5   Dose and Dose Constraints

The dose delivered to the chest wall is usually 50–50.4 Gy in 1.8–2 Gy fractions. Sometimes a 10–16 Gy boost to the mastectomy scar is added in high-risk patients, although there are minimal data about the benefit of a boost after mastectomy. The dose to the SCF is typically 45–50.4 Gy in 25–28 fractions. A 10–16 Gy boost should be considered for grossly involved nodes.

Although hypofractionated regimens have been used in the postmastectomy setting [1, 24], the risk of potential late toxicity, particularly brachial plexopathy and lymphedema, has limited its widespread use in the USA outside the setting of a clinical trial.

It is important to avoid high doses of radiation to the heart and lungs. While it seems prudent to minimize heart and lung dose to the greatest extent possible, the dose at which there becomes a clinically significant risk of heart and/or lung toxicity has not been reproducibly quantified. With this in mind, many institutions aim for a mean heart dose of <3 Gy and an ipsilateral lung V20 of <30%.

2.6   Special Considerations with Reconstruction

Patients who undergo immediate reconstruction at the time of mastectomy can pose additional challenges to treatment planning. Often, tissue expanders (TEs) will be placed under the pectoralis major muscle at the time of mastectomy and will be slowly inflated over several weeks, using weekly inflations of 50–100 cc of saline. This process allows the skin and muscle to be stretched in order to create a suitable pocket for the permanent implant. While some patients may be candidates for skin-sparing mastectomy that retains more of the skin envelope, many patients will have enough skin resected at the time of mastectomy such that the remaining skin will need to undergo expansion in order to fit the desired implant size. Since radiation therapy can produce a loss of skin elasticity, plastic surgeons typically will expand the ipsilateral side approximately 20% more than the intended implant size in order to compensate for potential contraction of the skin. Some plastic surgeons prefer that the radiotherapy be delivered with the TE in place, with the implant exchange occurring anywhere from 4 to 12 months after completion of radiotherapy. This sequence avoids direct irradiation of the permanent implant and allows for revision of the envelope at the time of permanent implant placement, although it delays the final surgical procedure for several months. From an oncologic standpoint, this may be a better approach for those with a very high risk of recurrence in order not to delay the radiotherapy treatment. Other plastic surgeons prefer completing the implant exchange prior to initiating radiotherapy as the wound healing may be better in unirradiated tissues [25, 26].

Treatment of the reconstructed breast with a temporary TE in place or with the permanent implant can create potential difficulty with the beam arrangements, dose distribution, and use of a bolus. Because of the uneven contour, the bolus may not conform perfectly to the chest wall. It may be useful to use in-vivo dosimeters (thermoluminescent dosimeter (TLD) or optically stimulated luminescent dosimeter (OSLD)) to ensure adequate dose to the skin.

When patients have bilateral TEs, one of the expanders may need to be partially deflated to improve the beam arrangement and dose distribution. The expansion could then be continued after completion of radiotherapy. This problem is more often significant for the contralateral expander. If the contralateral expander is expanded too much, treatment of the ipsilateral reconstructed breast can result in unintended dose to the contralateral side. Temporary deflation of the contralateral expander is often helpful.

Another challenge with treatment of a reconstructed breast with unilateral or bilateral TEs in place is the CT artifact from the internal metallic port (IMP) used

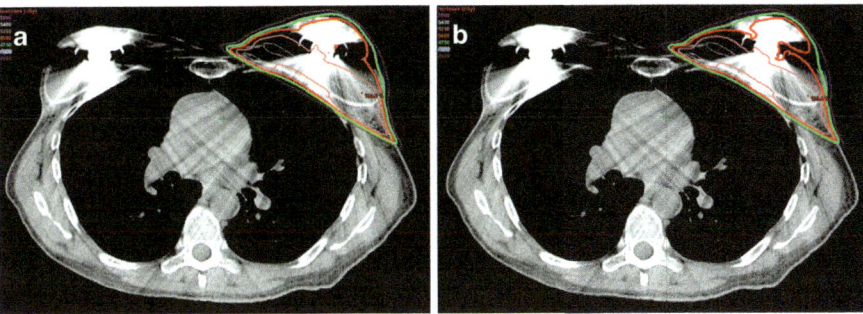

Fig. 2.6 Comparison of the dose distribution for patient with an internal metallic port (IMP): The treatment plan was generated using field-in-field technique and anisotropic analytical algorithm (AAA) (**a**). This plan then was recalculated using more accurate dose calculation algorithm, Acuros (**b**). Significant changes in target coverage along beam pathway through IMP and dose heterogeneity can be observed when comparing the plans

for injecting saline. This CT artifact can affect the dose calculations. This problem can usually be solved by contouring the IMP and assigning a Hounsfield unit (HU) corresponding to the type of material used for the port. Also, the areas of photon starvation and metal streaking are contoured and assigned HU of the soft tissue. Another way of eliminating the artifacts in the CT scan is to use artifact reduction software, which recently became commercially available by most CT vendors. Once the artifact reduction is performed, a more accurate dose calculation algorithm can be used, i.e., Acuros (Varian Medical Systems) or collapsed cone convolution superposition (Philips) (Fig. 2.6). Investigators have studied the effect of IMP on dose distribution around the port and have reported regions of underdose of up to 30 % in the area surrounding the IMP [27, 28]. More careful evaluation of treatment plans is warranted in these cases.

Reconstruction with autologous tissue can occur immediately at the time of mastectomy or be delayed until several months after completion of radiotherapy. With immediate reconstruction using autologous tissue, there may be fewer treatment planning challenges since the autologous tissue is generally less rigid than an inflated TE. Because the autologous tissue flaps often transfer abdominal skin to the chest, the bolus could be used over the entire tangent field or can be limited to the native chest wall skin. One main advantage of delayed reconstruction using autologous tissue is that the flap itself is not irradiated, potentially providing a better cosmetic outcome since an irradiated flap may contract and become more fibrotic over time.

Conclusions

PMRT is recommended for patients with four or more positive nodes or locally advanced disease. Some controversy remains regarding the benefit of PMRT in patients with T1-2 disease with 1–3 positive nodes or high-risk node-negative disease. Patients undergoing neoadjuvant chemotherapy followed by mastectomy should receive PMRT if they present with clinical stage III disease or have residual nodal involvement. The use of PMRT in those patients presenting with clinical stage II disease who achieve a pCR is currently under investigation.

With 3D CT-based treatment planning, the contouring of target volumes and normal structures, particularly the heart, lung, left ventricle, and left anterior descending artery, is critical to assure that improvements in breast cancer-specific survival are not offset by non-breast cancer mortality. CT-based treatment planning enables the use of several different techniques to achieve dose homogeneity and minimize dose to normal structures. Additional planning considerations may need to be taken into account for treatment of a reconstructed breast.

References

1. Ragaz J, Jackson SM, Le N et al (1997) Adjuvant radiotherapy and chemotherapy in node-positive premenopausal women with breast cancer. N Engl J Med 337:956–962
2. Overgaard M, Hansen PS, Overgaard J et al (1997) Postoperative radiotherapy in high-risk menopausal women with breast cancer who receive adjuvant chemotherapy. Danish Breast Cancer Cooperative Group 82b Trial. N Engl J Med 337:949–955
3. Overgaard M, Jensen MB, Overgaard J et al (1999) Postoperative radiotherapy in high-risk postmenopausal breast-cancer patients given adjuvant tamoxifen: Danish Breast Cancer Cooperative Group DBCG 82c randomized trial. Lancet 353:1641–1648
4. Clarke M, Collins R, Darby S et al (2005) Effects of radiotherapy and of differences in the extent of surgery for early breast cancer on local recurrence and 15-year survival: an overview of the randomized trials. Lancet 366:2087–2106
5. Early Breast Cancer Trialists' Collaborative Group (EBCTCG) (2014) Effect of radiotherapy after mastectomy and axillary surgery on 10-year recurrence and 20-year breast cancer mortality: meta-analysis of individual patient data for 8135 women in 22 randomised trials. Lancet 383:2127–2135
6. Harris JR, Halpin-Murphy P, McNeese M et al (1999) Consensus statement of postmastectomy radiation therapy. Int J Radiat Oncol Biol Phys 44:989–990
7. Recht A, Edge SB, Solin LJ et al (2001) Postmastectomy radiotherapy: guidelines of the American Society of Clinical Oncology. J Clin Oncol 19:1539–1569
8. Whelan TJ, Olivott IA, Parulekar WR et al (2015) Regional nodal irradiation in early-stage breast cancer. N Engl J Med 373(4):307–316
9. Poortmans PM, Collette S, Kirkove C et al (2015) Internal mammary and medial supraclavicular irradiation in breast cancer. N Engl J Med 373(4):317–327
10. SUPREMO. Selective use of postoperative radiotherapy after mastectomy (http://supremo-trial.com)
11. Kyndi M, Sorensen FB, Kndusen H et al (2008) Estrogen receptor, progesterone receptor, HER-2, and response to postmastectomy radiotherapy in high-risk breast cancer: the Danish Breast Cancer Cooperative Group. J Clin Oncol 26:1419–1426
12. Tseng YD, Uno H, Hughes ME et al (2015) Biological subtype predicts risk of locoregional recurrence after mastectomy and impact of postmastectomy radiation in a large national database. Int J Radiat Oncol Biol Phys 93(3):622–630
13. Buchholz TA, Katz A, Strom EA et al (2002) Pathologic tumor size and lymph node status predict for different rates of locoregional recurrence after mastectomy for breast cancer patients treated with neoadjuvant versus adjuvant chemotherapy. Int J Radiat Oncol Biol Phys 53:880–888
14. Buchholz TA, Tucker SL, Masullo L et al (2002) Predictors of local-regional recurrence after neoadjuvant chemotherapy and mastectomy without radiation. J Clin Oncol 20:17–23

15. McGuire SE, Gonzalez-Angulo AM, Huang EH et al (2007) Postmastectomy radiation improves the outcomes of patients with locally advanced breast cancer who achieve a pathologic complete response to neoadjuvant chemotherapy. Int J Radiat Oncol Biol Phys 68:1004–1009

16. Mamounas EP, Anderson SJ, Dignam JJ et al (2012) Predictors of locoregional recurrence after neoadjuvant chemotherapy: results from combined analysis of National Surgical Adjuvant Breast and Bowel Project B-18 and B-27. J Clin Oncol 30:3960–3966

17. Buchholz TA, Lehman CD, Harris JR et al (2008) Statement of the science concerning locoregional treatments after preoperative chemotherapy for breast cancer: a National Cancer Institute conference. J Clin Oncol 26:791–797

18. National Surgical Adjuvant Breast and Bowel Project (NSABP). NSABP B-51/RTOG 1304 (http://www.nsabp.pitt.edu/B-51.asp)

19. RTOG. Breast cancer atlas for radiation therapy planning: consensus definitions (https://www.rtog.org/CoreLab/ContouringAtlases/BreastCancerAtlas.aspx)

20. Offersen BV, Boersma LJ, Kirkove C et al (2015) ESTRO consensus guideline on target volume delineation for elective radiation therapy of early stage breast cancer. Radiother Oncol 114:3–10

21. Moran MS, Haffty BG (2009) Radiation techniques and toxicities for locally advanced breast cancer. Semin Radiat Oncol 19:244–255

22. Daves I, Rumble RB, Bowen J et al (2012) Intensity-modulated radiotherapy in the treatment of breast cancer. Clin Oncol 24(7):488–498

23. Hall EJ, Wuu C-S (2003) Radiation-induced second cancers: the impact of 3D-CRT and IMRT. Int J Radiat Oncol Biol Phys 56:83–88

24. Haviland JS, Owen JR, Dewar JA et al (2013) The UK Standardisation of Breast Radiotherapy (START) trials of radiotherapy hypofractionation for treatment of early breast cancer: 10-year follow-up results of two randomized controlled trials. Lancet Oncol 14:1086–1094

25. Cordeiro PG, Albornoz CR, McCormick B et al (2015) What is the optimum timing of postmastectomy radiotherapy in two-stage prosthetic reconstruction: radiation to the tissue expander or permanent implant? Plast Reconstr Surg 135(6):1509–1517

26. El-Sabawi B, Carey JN, Hagopian TM et al (2016) Radiation and breast reconstruction: algorithmic approach and evidence-based outcomes. J Surg Oncol. doi:10.1002/jso.24143 [Epub ahead of print]

27. Thompson R, Morgan AM (2005) Investigation into dosimetric effect of a MAGNA-SITE™ tissue expander on post-mastectomy radiotherapy. Med Phys 32:1640–1646

28. Chen SA, Ogunleye T, Dhabbaan A, Huang EH, Losken A, Gabram S, Davis L, Torres MA (2013) Impact of internal metallic ports in temporary tissue expanders on postmastectomy radiation dose distribution. Int J Radiat Oncol Biol Phys 85(3):630–635

Techniques for Internal Mammary Node Radiation

3

Jean Wright, Sook Kien Ng, and Oren Cahlon

Content

The clinical decision to include the internal mammary (IM) nodal chain into radiation treatment fields for breast cancer is complex, and the literature surrounding this decision is controversial and even conflicting [1–5]. However, with three recent high profile publications supporting the use of IM radiation even in relatively low-risk women, there will likely be an increasing trend toward IM radiation in the coming years [6]. The primary reasons not to treat these nodes are that it can be technically challenging and may increase exposure to the heart, lung, and contralateral breast. Ultimately, the decision to treat the IM nodes for an individual patient balances the estimated clinical benefit based on the patient's scenario with the potential additional toxicity that may be conferred by treating this nodal group. This chapter will focus on the various techniques that may be employed to treat the IM nodes, rather than the complex decision-making involved for an individual patient.

Several early publications compared techniques for post-mastectomy radiation (PMRT) and evaluated the different approaches with respect to chest wall and IM

J. Wright (✉) • S.K. Ng
Department of Radiation Oncology and Molecular Radiation Sciences,
Johns Hopkins University, Baltimore, MD, USA
e-mail: jeanwright@jhmi.edu

O. Cahlon
Department of Radiation Oncology, Memorial Sloan Kettering Cancer Center,
New York, NY, USA

© Springer International Publishing Switzerland 2016
J.R. Bellon et al. (eds.), *Radiation Therapy Techniques and Treatment Planning for Breast Cancer*, Practical Guides in Radiation Oncology,
DOI 10.1007/978-3-319-40392-2_3

coverage as well as the heart and lung dose [7, 8]. The two general techniques that emerged from these comparisons as providing the best IM coverage with relative sparing of the heart and lung, broadly categorized, were electron or electron/photon fields matched to shallow photon tangents and partially wide photon tangents. Two other emerging techniques for IM radiation have recently garnered attention, both developed primarily to improve IM coverage: proton therapy and intensity modulated radiation/volumetric modulated arc therapy (IMRT/VMAT).

Regardless of the specific technique used, the first step in all cases is to clearly identify the target. Institutions vary in their implementation of contouring the breast or chest wall for treatment planning, but in the current era, it is critical, at a minimum, to contour the nodal targets. The current RTOG atlas for breast cancer (readily accessible at www.rtog.org/CoreLab/ContouringAtlases/BreastCancerAtlas. aspx) details the internal mammary chain anatomy. Generally, one contours the internal mammary artery and vein, which are almost always visible on a simple non-contrast planning CT, and considers this as the IM clinical target volume (CTV). The extent of IM coverage one chooses may vary with the clinical scenario. The IM nodes sitting in the first through third intercostal spaces are the most common and high-value target used in the MA.20 study [2], but in certain settings, such as a lower inner quadrant tumor and/or multiple high-risk features, one may choose to include the first through fifth intercostal spaces, as was done in the EORTC 22922 study [1]. Two other structures that must be contoured in all cases are the heart and the lungs, which are the critical organs at risk (OAR) in breast cancer treatment planning. Once contouring is complete, one is ready to begin planning and selecting the optimal technique for an individual patient.

The simplest and most accessible technique for IM coverage is likely the partially wide tangent [9]. This approach relies on a modification of the standard photon approach that is commonly used in the setting of radiation to the intact breast without regional nodal radiation and implements only two beam angles with modified blocking. In general, if one has chosen to include the IM nodes, the undissected axillary and supraclavicular nodes are typically also included. However, because the match line between the supraclavicular field and the photon tangents is generally set at the caudal border of the clavicle, the first contoured IM nodes sit below this match and are included in the breast or chest wall tangent photon fields. Thus, a traditional mono-isocentric technique may be used.

In the case of partially wide tangents, the posterior field border is placed deeply enough that the contoured internal mammary nodes are covered in the fields. This results in fields that would include an uncomfortably high volume of the heart and lung in the fields if not further modified. Thus, blocking is then added to conform to the shape of the contoured IM target, with an often sharp indentation just below the IM nodes to spare the heart and lung below the inferior-most IM contour. The anatomic location of this inferior-most IM contour in relation to the heart will vary with individual anatomy, as well as the extent of IM coverage that is chosen. For many patients, when the first through third intercostal spaces are targeted, the inferior border sits above the cardiac contour allowing for cardiac sparing. However, for cases when the IM chain extends to the level of the heart, it is very difficult to cover

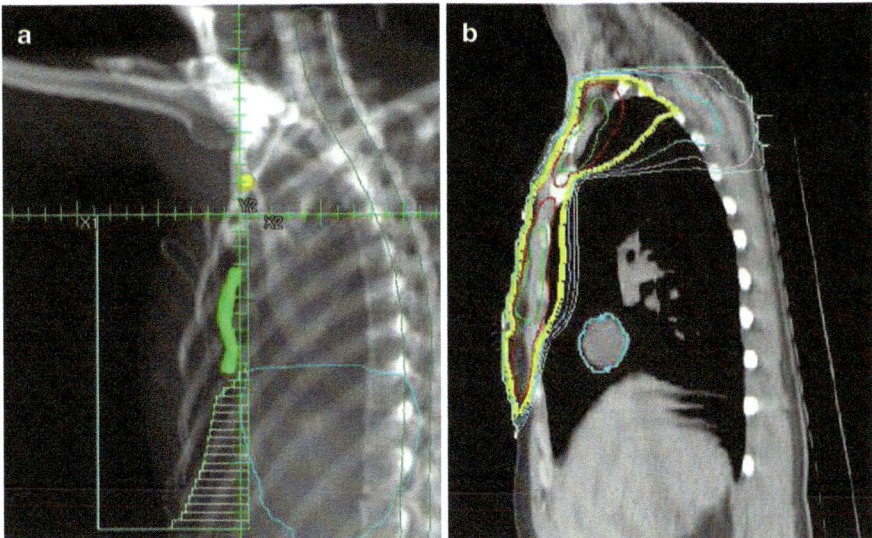

Fig. 3.1 Partially wide tangents. Figure (**a**) shows a digitally reconstructed radiograph (DRR) of a medial tangent beam, with the posterior edge placed deep to the internal mammary (IM) node contour in *green*. Below the IM contour, the field is blocked to shield the heart, silhouetted in *blue*, and to conform to the wired breast contour. Note the sharp indentation of the field below the IM contour. Figure (**b**) shows the related isodose lines in sagittal projection. The *yellow line* represents the 90 % isodose line (IDL)

the inferior portion without giving excessive dose to the heart. In these cases, many clinicians will simply omit the lower portion of the IM chain from the field or opt for an alternate technique. Figures 3.1 and 3.2 depict a representative partially wide tangent plan.

The second common technique for coverage of the IM nodes is medial electron field(s) matched to shallow photon tangents. This technique is also widely accessible, as standard linear accelerators have both electron and photon capabilities, but is somewhat more complex in that it requires field matching between two different modalities. Though more complex, this approach can be readily learned and adopted with proper attention to key planning and setup details.

Once the targets and OAR have been contoured, the first beam to place is generally the medial electron beam, followed by the medial photon tangent. With this approach, a bit of "trial-and-error" is necessary – first placing the electron beam, then the medial tangent, and then adjusting back and forth to optimize the match.

One begins with the electron beam, placed at a straight AP or zero degree angle. To place this beam, one uses a unique isocenter in the center of the proposed field, on the skin surface since electrons are typically treated with an SSD technique. In the setting of a relatively flat target, such as the chest wall with no reconstruction or a deflated expander or breast tissue that naturally flattens with gravity in the supine position, the tissue depth is quite even from the medial to lateral edges of the

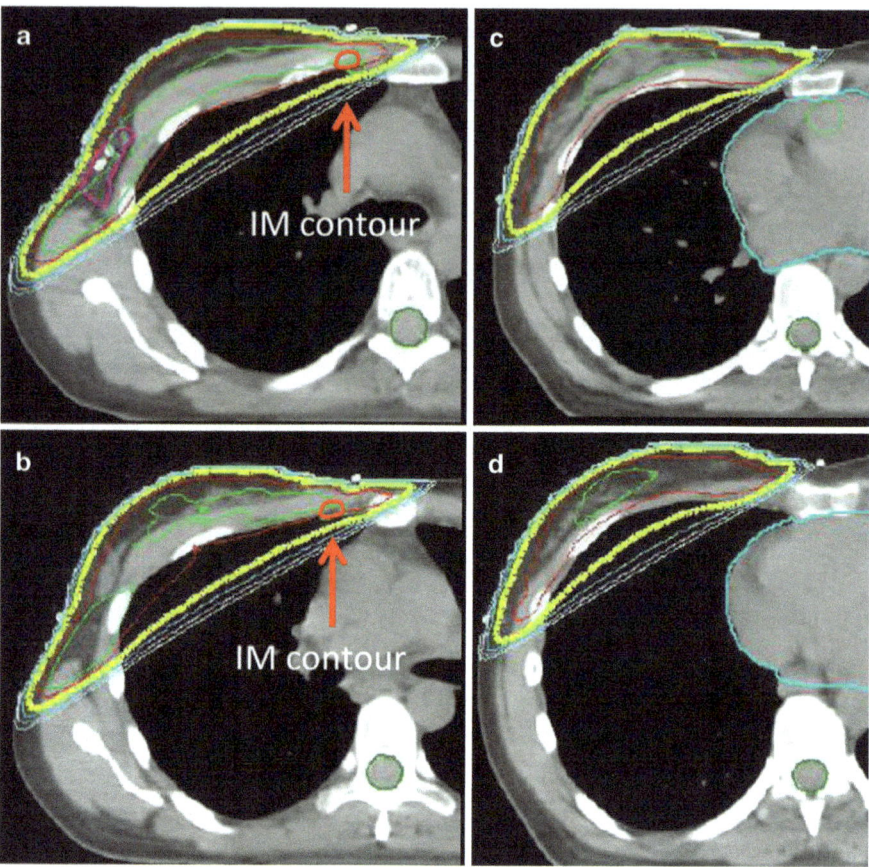

Fig. 3.2 Partially wide tangents. Figure depicts the axial CT images related to the DRR shown in Fig. 3.1. (**a**) Is the superior-most contour, with *yellow* again representing the 90 % IDL. Note that the low axilla, contoured in *pink* and identified with clips in this image, is included in this tangent beam, as well as the IM contour in *red*; both are covered by the 90 % IDL. (**b–d**) Move sequentially inferior, with tighter blocking and less lung in images **c** and **d** which are below the IM contour

electron field. The most even dose distribution would be achieved at this zero angle, as shown in Fig. 3.3, so one begins with this "ideal" electron beam, with a minimum field width of about 4 cm for optimal electron dosimetry, and placed such that the medial border provides adequate margin on the contoured IM nodes.

Second, one places the medial tangent using the same isocenter as the supraclavicular field ("mono-isocentric" technique) – one may need to adjust the position of this isocenter and alter the supraclavicular field later. The medial border of the tangent should be lateral enough to avoid contact with the heart and should be angled similarly to a standard tangent to cover the breast or chest wall target. This typically results in very shallow tangent beams with no more than 1 cm of the lung on the DRR and an electron field that treats the IM nodes and the medial portion of the chest wall.

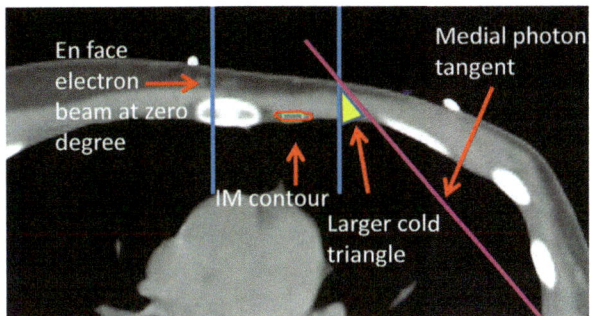

Fig. 3.3 Figure depicts an initial setup for a medial electron beam matched to photon tangents. Note that the direct en face electron beam at a 0° angle results in a very even tissue depth across the field but that the skin surface match to the photon tangent beam results in a relatively large "cold triangle." This setup, therefore, is a good starting place but requires additional beam angling to optimize the setup

Once these basic fields are placed, one can begin to make adjustments. The electron beam will need to be angled; the optimal angle will vary from patient to patient but is generally between 15° and 30° away from the straight AP field and between 5° and 15° rotated from the medial tangent. There are two factors that contribute to choosing the optimal angle for a given patient: the variability in the depth of the electron field and the size of the "cold triangle" that results from an imperfect match with the medial photon tangent. While the AP electron beam angle minimizes tissue depth variability, a large "cold triangle" results when matched to photon tangents that are adequately angled to spare the heart and lung, as shown in Fig. 3.3. To minimize this cold triangle between the electron and photon fields, one might angle the electron field sharply to create a seamless match with the photon tangent. However, this results in significant variability in tissue depth across the field, impairing the dosimetric result. The optimal beam angles, then, balance the desire to have a uniform field depth with the need to minimize the size of the cold triangle. A rule of thumb would be that the angle between the electron and photon fields should range from 5° to 15°, as shown in Fig. 3.4. As the electron field is rotated toward the medial tangent field, the hot spot of the plan also typically increases. The hot spot in these plans is usually in the medial portion of the tangent field and is created by the bowing out of the lower isodose lines of the electron field into the medial tangent. The hot spots in these plans often reach 130 % of the prescribed dose. Figure 3.5 depicts isodose curves on axial images derived from the beam arrangement shown in Fig. 3.4.

Once the field angles are chosen, one can begin to focus on the details of the electron-photon match. In a standard-risk patient, the match may be placed directly on the skin surface. There are certain scenarios in which one might consider overlapping the match by 3–5 mm. In a particularly high-risk patient, such as one with inflammatory breast cancer, dosimetric coverage should be prioritized, and a small overlap is appropriate. One might also consider overlap if the high-risk area of the target – such as lumpectomy cavity, or known margin positivity – is located at the

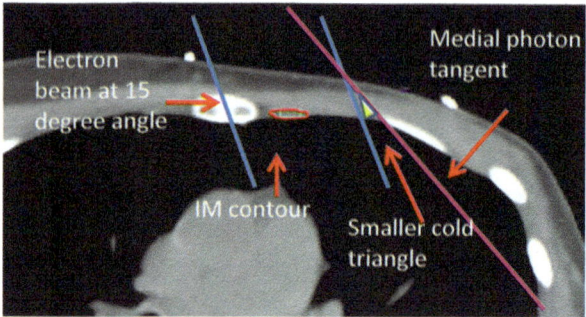

Fig. 3.4 Figure depicts the same patient as Fig. 3.3, but this time the electron beam is angled 15°, resulting in only minimal variation in the tissue depth across the field. Still matching at the skin surface, the resultant cold triangle is smaller than that shown in Fig. 3.3. This image represents a beam arrangement that is ready for dosimetric planning

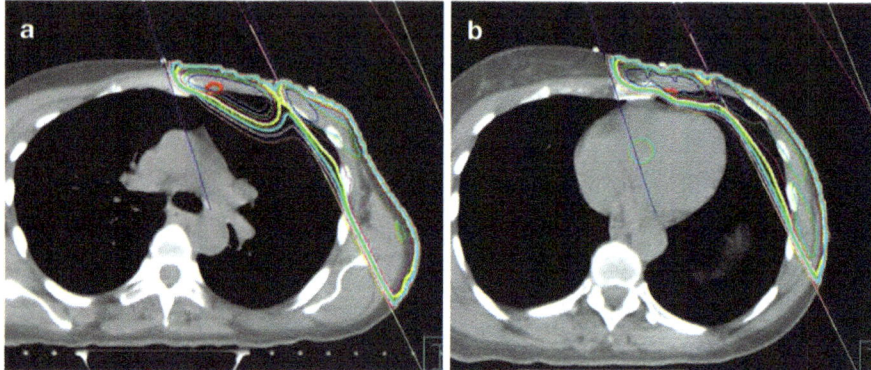

Fig. 3.5 Figure shows the resultant isodose curves related to the beam arrangement shown in Fig. 3.4. (**a**) Depicts a small cold area at the match; note that the *turquoise line*, which represents the 80 % IDL, covers the full area including the cold triangle. (**b**) Depicts the isodose lines at the level of the heart, demonstrating how this technique can be used to sculpt the radiation dose around the heart in a curvilinear manner

match. In the current era, feathering is not considered necessary unless significant overlap is planned, even if a breath hold technique is used. Toggling between the axial CT images, DRRs, and skin renderings allows the planner to visualize the match and make minor adjustments to tailor the match line from top to bottom of the fields.

Finally, once these basic parameters are set, the planner can attend to dosimetry details such as electron and photon beam energy and the correct prescription iso-dose line. Again, minor field adjustments will likely be made even at this phase of planning. Some institutions divide the IM electron field into a superior and an infe-rior field and use a higher electron energy superiorly where IM coverage is priori-tized and a lower electron energy inferiorly to better spare the heart [10]. Typically 9–12 MeV electrons are used for good coverage of the IM chain. In larger women,

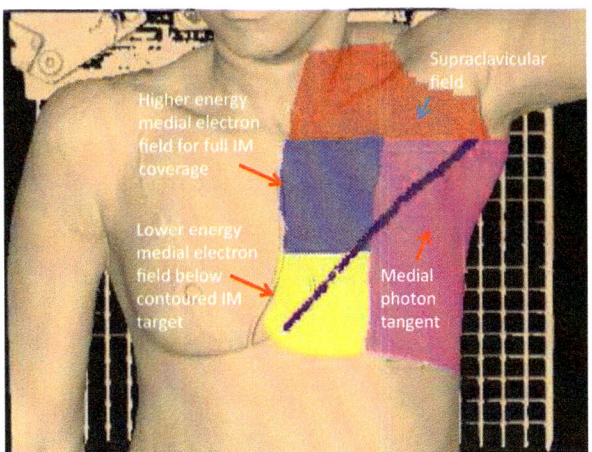

Fig. 3.6 Figure depicts the skin rendering from a complex plan that matches two electron fields with a supraclavicular field and photon tangents. The superior electron field is higher energy, designed to cover the IM contour, and the lower electron field is of a lower energy, designed to cover the chest wall more superficially. Note the skin surface matching of the various fields. This demonstrates how a skin rendering can be very useful to evaluate how a complex beam arrangement comes together on the patient

the IM nodes can lie at 5 cm depth or more below the skin surface, requiring higher energy electrons. Rarely, it may be appropriate to supplement the electron field with a very low-weighted photon beam (perhaps 5 monitor units) to improve the depth of coverage. Caution is needed when using photons or higher energy electrons as they will deliver more dose to the lung and possibly also the heart. In such cases, a different technique might be preferred. Figure 3.6 depicts a skin rendering modeling the matching of an upper and a lower electron field to photon tangents. It is essential in the setting of matched fields that the physician evaluates the light fields on the patient in the treatment room as a part of the initial setup, to ensure the matching is carried out as planned. Bolus is not typically needed for the electron field because electrons deliver high skin doses; however, bolus can be used over the whole field or parts of the field as a tissue compensator to pull dose out of the lung. Caution is warranted with the use of a tissue compensator, as this does increase skin dose and can result in long-term telangiectatic skin changes.

Proton therapy is another emerging technique in breast cancer, particularly useful for patients who require IM treatment [11, 12]. When treating the IM nodes as part of comprehensive regional nodal irradiation, proton therapy is able to achieve excellent target coverage and maintain very low heart and lung doses. Protons also result in a homogenous dose distribution with few hot and cold spots (Fig. 3.7). Contouring for proton therapy is similar to photon therapy, but because a proton plan will only deliver dose to contoured targets, the full breast or chest wall must also be contoured. Because of this difference, there are unique contouring guidelines for proton therapy, and these can be found at https://www.rtog.org/CoreLab/ContouringAtlases/RADCOMPBreastAtlas.aspx. Patients are simulated in a

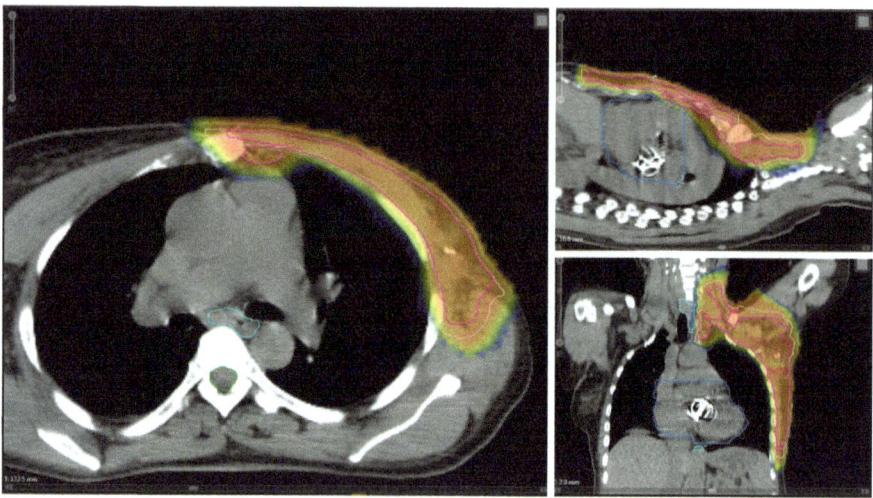

Fig. 3.7 Isodose distributions for a proton plan in axial, sagittal, and coronal views. Proton plans such as this generally achieve mean heart doses of about 1 Gy, V20 of the ipsilateral lung of about 15 %, and V5 of the ipsilateral lung of about 35 %

similar fashion to photons and electrons (Alpha Cradle, breast board), although it is also possible to treat patients with the arms down if needed with proton therapy. With uniform scanning or passive scattering, two matching anterior oblique fields (chest wall field matched to a supraclavicular fossa field) are used. The match line is feathered. Daily image guidance is recommended and typically done with 2dKV imaging and/or surface imaging such as AlignRT. Pencil beam scanning (PBS) is now becoming more commonly used and has several advantages over uniform scanning/passive scattering, including treatment with a single field (avoiding match lines, feathering, hot/cold spots), faster treatment delivery, and skin sparing, if desired. Proton therapy is not widely available and is currently being compared to standard techniques in a randomized trial, RADCOMP. Details are available at https://clinicaltrials.gov/ct2/show/NCT02603341. The RADCOMP trial will specifically be enrolling patients who require IM irradiation and randomize them to proton vs non-proton techniques, comparing late effects of treatment. It remains to be seen if the dosimetric benefits of proton therapy will translate to clinical gains, and at this time the approach remains a technique that is only available at limited centers with access to proton therapy.

Another technique that may be used is multifield intensity modulated radiation/volumetric modulated arc therapy (IMRT/VMAT). This approach offers excellent target coverage with improved homogeneity and high-dose conformality but comes at the expense of a "low-dose" bath with the 5–10 Gy isodose lines covering large portions of the thorax, including the heart. Due to this cardiac exposure, this approach is not favored by many clinicians despite the other appealing dosimetric features. It is generally not possible to meet the cardiac parameters described below with this approach, but this technique may be suitable for a high-risk patient where coverage is key and late effects are a lower concern.

Regardless of technique, the same basic dosimetric objectives should apply. In breast cancer treatment planning, there are no standardized target coverage or OAR parameters. However, we may look to current RTOG trials to provide guidance; RTOG 1304 specifically evaluates the impact of nodal coverage in node-positive breast cancer patients who convert to node-negative after preoperative chemotherapy and is an excellent resource for dosimetric guidelines. In the protocol, one expands the contoured IM nodal CTV by 5 mm in medial, lateral, superior, and inferior dimensions to an IM planning target volume (PTV), with a coverage goal of 90% of the IM PTV receiving 90% of the prescribed dose. Outside of a protocol, many would omit the PTV expansion and aim for 90% of the prescribed dose covering 100% of the contoured IM CTV. Similarly, outside of a protocol, one may evaluate the 90% isodose line (IDL) on the axial CT images and ensure coverage of the breast or chest wall target in this manner. Particularly with the matched electron-photon technique, the dose volume histogram (DVH) view of the breast or chest wall target may appear suboptimal due to hot spots at the surface match and the cold triangle below this. A rule of thumb for the cold triangle is that the dose in the triangle should be no less than 70% of the prescribed dose. Outside of a clinical trial, many clinicians rely on evaluating the visual coverage of the 90% isodose line on the axial CT images rather than the DVH.

One must balance the above coverage goals with doses to OAR, particularly the heart. Again, there are no standardized parameters for OAR in breast cancer, and the primary objective should be to achieve doses that are as low as reasonably achievable. RTOG 1304 specifies that for those receiving comprehensive nodal radiation, the mean heart dose should be ≤4 Gy, though many institutions aim for 3 Gy or even less. For left-sided cases, ≤5% of the contoured heart should receive 25 Gy or more, and ≤30% should receive 15 Gy or more, while for right-sided cases, 0% of the contoured heart should receive 25 Gy, and 10% should receive 15 Gy or more. Again, lower doses than this are desirable if this can be reasonably achieved. A recent literature review showed great variability in cardiac doses published in studies from 2003 to 2103, demonstrating the lack of consensus on cardiac constraints [13].

Strict cardiac dose constraints are often difficult to meet while achieving strong target coverage. A publication from MD Anderson reviewing actual IM doses delivered at their institution, when retrospectively contoured based on the RTOG atlas, showed that with 3D conformal radiation techniques, the mean V90 of the IM contour was actually 80%. For a 5 mm expansion of the contour to a PTV, the V90 would be significantly lower [14]. Thus, the clinician is often faced with balancing achieving target coverage and keeping OAR doses below tolerance. Often compromises are needed and must be made based on many individual factors for a specific patient such as comorbidities, age, risk of disease, and identifying high- and low-risk target areas. The MD Anderson publication is comforting in demonstrating that excellent local control is achieved with traditional 3D conformal techniques, despite compromised target volume coverage compared to current RTOG trial standards.

The presence of a reconstruction may influence which of these techniques is best suited to a particular patient. The electron-photon technique works best in the setting of a relatively flat chest wall or intact breast tissue or autologous reconstruction that does not arise steeply from the chest wall. Because of the variability in tissue thickness when an inflated expander or implant is in place, the dosimetry with an electron beam can be markedly impaired compared to a flat chest wall. In this setting, the partially wide tangent technique is often better suited. Alternatively, one may deflate a tissue expander to allow for the use of the electron-photon technique.

Deep inspiration breath hold (DIBH) techniques, described elsewhere in this textbook, are also commonly used in the setting of planned IM coverage to improve dosimetric outcomes, particularly for the heart. The combination of matched electron-photon fields with DIBH results in particularly favorable dosimetry but is more challenging to implement. The principles of the technique are the same as described above, but greater attention is needed to ensure appropriate matching of the fields in the treatment room. Increasing the number of fields with DIBH also increases the time needed for treatment. This greater effort and time commitment pays off in terms of dosimetry but is only superior to more standard techniques if the treatment planners and, critically, the therapy staff have experience and comfort with this approach. One might consider a stepwise implementation of this approach, gradually increasing complexity to the point where the best balance between dosimetry and reproducible treatment delivery at one's institution is achieved.

Each of the techniques described above has advantages and disadvantages. The partially wide tangent technique is the simplest to deliver and is excellent for patients who have undergone immediate tissue expander/implant reconstruction because it is less sensitive to the depth of the chest wall. One of the disadvantages is the inability to shape the higher isodose lines around the target, resulting in higher lung doses than the other techniques. It is also difficult to cover the superior portion of the IM chain in the tangent fields without significant increases in lung dose. This technique can be relatively easily incorporated with DIBH, which can significantly reduce cardiac exposure. The electron/photon technique is a more technically challenging technique but generally results in lower lung doses due to the rapid dose falloff of the electrons. This is particularly true in cases in which the chest wall is relatively thin, and higher energy electrons can be avoided. There is more dose heterogeneity overall with these plans, resulting in significant cold and hot spots. The use of DIBH is much more challenging with this technique. Proton therapy offers optimal dosimetry with the ability to sculpt the high-dose region around the target and without the low-dose exposure. The major disadvantage of proton therapy is the lack of access with only about 20 operational centers currently, as well as the high cost of treatment. IMRT/VMAT offers excellent target coverage with improved homogeneity and the ability to better sculpt the higher isodose lines off the target. This comes at the expense of a "low-dose" bath with the 5–10 Gy lines covering large portions of the thorax.

The best technique for a given patient will thus depend on multiple factors including patient anatomy (including presence and type of reconstruction in mastectomy patients), extent of IM coverage that is planned, available technology, and the treatment team's comfort with the various techniques. There is no one approach that is superior overall, and the details of treatment planning are another opportunity in breast cancer management for tailoring treatment to each patient's unique scenario.

References

1. Poortmans PM, Collette S, Kirkove C et al (2015) Internal mammary and medial supraclavicular irradiation in breast cancer. N Engl J Med 373:317–327
2. Whelan TJ, Olivotto IA, Parulekar WR et al (2015) Regional nodal irradiation in early-stage breast cancer. N Engl J Med 373:307–316
3. Thorsen LB, Offersen BV, Dano H et al (2016) DBCG-IMN: a population-based cohort study on the effect of internal mammary node irradiation in early node-positive breast cancer. J Clin Oncol 34:314–320
4. Hennequin C, Bossard N, Servagi-Vernat S et al (2013) Ten-year survival results of a randomized trial of irradiation of internal mammary nodes after mastectomy. Int J Radiat Oncol Biol Phys 86:860–866
5. McGale P, Taylor C, Correa C et al (2014) Effect of radiotherapy after mastectomy and axillary surgery on 10-year recurrence and 20-year breast cancer mortality: meta-analysis of individual patient data for 8135 women in 22 randomised trials. Lancet 383:2127–2135
6. Haffty BG, Whelan T, Poortmans PM (2016) Radiation of the internal mammary nodes: is there a benefit? J Clin Oncol 34:297–299
7. Pierce LJ, Butler JB, Martel MK et al (2002) Postmastectomy radiotherapy of the chest wall: dosimetric comparison of common techniques. Int J Radiat Oncol Biol Phys 52:1220–1230
8. Arthur DW, Arnfield MR, Warwicke LA et al (2000) Internal mammary node coverage: an investigation of presently accepted techniques. Int J Radiat Oncol Biol Phys 48:139–146
9. Marks LB, Hebert ME, Bentel G et al (1994) To treat or not to treat the internal mammary nodes: a possible compromise. Int J Radiat Oncol Biol Phys 29:903–909
10. Oh JL, Buchholz TA (2009) Internal mammary node radiation: a proposed technique to spare cardiac toxicity. J Clin Oncol 27:e172–e173; author reply e174.
11. Depauw N, Batin E, Daartz J et al (2015) A novel approach to postmastectomy radiation therapy using scanned proton beams. Int J Radiat Oncol Biol Phys 91:427–434
12. Cuaron JJ, Chon B, Tsai H et al (2015) Early toxicity in patients treated with postoperative proton therapy for locally advanced breast cancer. Int J Radiat Oncol Biol Phys 92:284–291
13. Taylor CW, Wang Z, Macaulay E et al (2015) Exposure of the heart in breast cancer radiation therapy: a systematic review of heart doses published during 2003 to 2013. Int J Radiat Oncol Biol Phys 93:845–853
14. Fontanilla HP, Woodward WA, Lindberg ME et al (2012) Current clinical coverage of Radiation Therapy Oncology Group-defined target volumes for postmastectomy radiation therapy. Pract Radiat Oncol 2:201–209

Target Delineation and Contouring

4

Kimberly S. Corbin and Robert W. Mutter

Contents

4.1 Introduction

Adjuvant whole breast radiotherapy (RT) reduces the risk of recurrence and improves survival after breast-conserving surgery [1]. Recently, the addition of radiation to the high axillary, supraclavicular, and internal mammary lymph nodes has been shown to result in further reductions in locoregional and distant relapse and improvements in disease-free survival [2, 3]. In women with lymph node-positive breast cancer, postmastectomy RT to the chest wall and regional lymph nodes improves overall survival [4]. These established benefits of breast cancer RT are accompanied by an increased risk of delayed morbidity, such as lymphedema [5], secondary malignancy [6], and major coronary events [7]. Therefore, meticulous treatment planning is needed in order to optimize the therapeutic ratio in patients with indications for RT [8].

K.S. Corbin • R.W. Mutter (✉)
Department of Radiation Oncology, Mayo Clinic, Rochester, MN, USA
e-mail: Mutter.robert@mayo.edu

© Springer International Publishing Switzerland 2016
J.R. Bellon et al. (eds.), *Radiation Therapy Techniques and Treatment Planning for Breast Cancer*, Practical Guides in Radiation Oncology,
DOI 10.1007/978-3-319-40392-2_4

Treatment planning for breast cancer RT has changed significantly in recent years. The two-dimensional era, in which bony landmarks were used to define RT fields, relied on uniform prescription depths. However, anatomical variation in the depths and locations of nodal regions resulted in suboptimal target coverage [9–11]. Two-dimensional planning has largely been supplanted by three-dimensional (3D) techniques, in which patient-specific anatomical clinical target volumes (CTVs) are defined by cross-sectional computerized tomography (CT) scans. As part of this transition, several groups proposed contouring guidelines and atlases in order to reduce physician-to-physician inconsistencies in CTV delineation and to prepare for the adoption of CTV-based planning in clinical trials [12–15]. Evidence suggests that the use of contouring guidelines does reduce variability in treatment planning. However, even among experts and across guidelines, there remain discrepancies in recommendations for the delineation of CTVs and organs at risk [16–18].

One reason for the discrepancy is that when traditional fields are applied to contoured CTVs, suboptimal coverage of the defined targets and/or higher doses to critical structures may ensue [19–21]. Because of the excellent locoregional control achieved with RT as part of combined modality therapy for breast cancer prior to the emergence of CTV-based planning, some have raised caution regarding the potential impact of larger treatment volumes with CTV-based planning [12, 21]. In contrast, improvements in locoregional and distant disease control have recently been observed in selected patients with more comprehensive nodal targeting. These results highlighted that clinically significant locoregional disease may go undetected or be detected only after distant relapse occurs, raising the possibility that better coverage of areas truly at risk of harboring microscopic disease could further enhance treatment outcomes in some high-risk patients [2, 3, 20, 22–24]. With conventional breast cancer field design, a considerable amount of tissue in the axillary and supraclavicular regions outside of the breast/chest wall and nodal CTVs, as defined by some consensus guidelines, can receive a significant fraction of the prescription dose due to the gradual attenuation of x-rays passing through the tissue [25–27]. Recently, more conformal techniques such as proton therapy and intensity-modulated radiotherapy (IMRT) are being employed for the treatment of breast cancer. These newer technologies may actually result in unintentional "sparing" of some areas at risk which were previously covered by traditional fields [24, 26, 28]. Target volume definition theoretically should not differ between techniques, yet accurate delineation may be of greater importance with more conformal approaches. Therefore, modern breast cancer RT practice requires an advanced understanding of patient anatomy and locations of areas at highest risk of harboring microscopic disease in order to inform CTV delineation and provide the best opportunity to optimize the therapeutic ratio.

It is within this context that a burgeoning literature has emerged, studying patterns of disease spread with cross-sectional imaging and using an evidence-based approach to reexamine guidelines that emerged early in the transition to CTV-based planning [29–31, 42]. Herein, we review this literature and propose a framework for target volume delineation. We propose that a "one-size-fits-all" approach to breast cancer CTVs is inadequate and highlight areas where CTVs should reasonably be tailored based on the specific clinical and pathologic risk profile of individual patients. This chapter focuses on recommendations for patients undergoing adjuvant radiotherapy to address potential sites of residual microscopic disease and describes potential scenarios where patients with gross disease or recurrence may require more comprehensive volumes. We have also included a Contouring Atlas (Fig. 4.2a–p) and a table emphasizing recommended modifications to the historical RTOG consensus volumes.

4.2   Axillary Node Targets

The axilla is the primary site of lymphatic spread from the breast [32]. Importantly, traditional surgical landmarks used to separate the axilla into levels 1–3 are not truly "anatomical," as the pathways of spread to each level are not distinct (unlike other disease sites such as the head and neck) and no true barrier exists between them. The breast's lymphatic pathways originate from interlobular connective tissue and communicate with subcutaneous networks [32]. The primary breast lymphatic flow is around the inferior border of the pectoralis major muscle and into the anterior pectoral group of nodes located behind that muscle. However, additional accessory pathways exist. These accessory routes can result in direct spread to lymph nodes in the more posterior aspects of the axilla, interpectoral, and apical axillary regions, along with the infraclavicular, supraclavicular, and parasternal (internal mammary) sites [32]. Thus, for those with risk of lymph node involvement, all regions of the axilla may be considered as potential sites for harboring microscopic disease. Recently, the addition of high axillary RT (along with supraclavicular and internal mammary lymph node RT) to whole breast irradiation has been shown to improve outcomes in early-stage breast cancer [2, 3, 23]. In addition, axillary lymph node dissection is increasingly omitted following a positive sentinel lymph node biopsy in patients with early-stage breast cancer who will be undergoing adjuvant radiotherapy [25, 33]. Therefore, accurate delineation of the axillary CTV is critical in the modern breast cancer radiotherapy practice.

Key anatomic structures used to define the regions are the pectoralis major, the pectoralis minor, the serratus anterior, the latissimus dorsi, the teres minor, the teres major, the subscapular, and the axillary vessels [32]. The RTOG has proposed consensus definitions for target volume delineation in breast cancer radiation therapy planning [15]. The accuracy of these guidelines for coverage of involved lymph nodes has been examined. MacDonald et al. used lymphotropic nanoparticle-enhanced MRI for lymph node mapping in breast cancer patients with pathologic correlates [34]. The RTOG guidelines were used for contouring, and the inclusion of pathologically involved nodes within the contours was examined. Eighty-two percent of malignant lymph nodes were included within the volume. Lymph nodes outside of the target volumes were most often located anterior to the line connecting the pectoralis major muscle and the latissimus dorsi (Fig. 4.1a). While this region is not covered by the RTOG atlas, it is included in other proposed anatomical based contouring guidelines [12, 35].

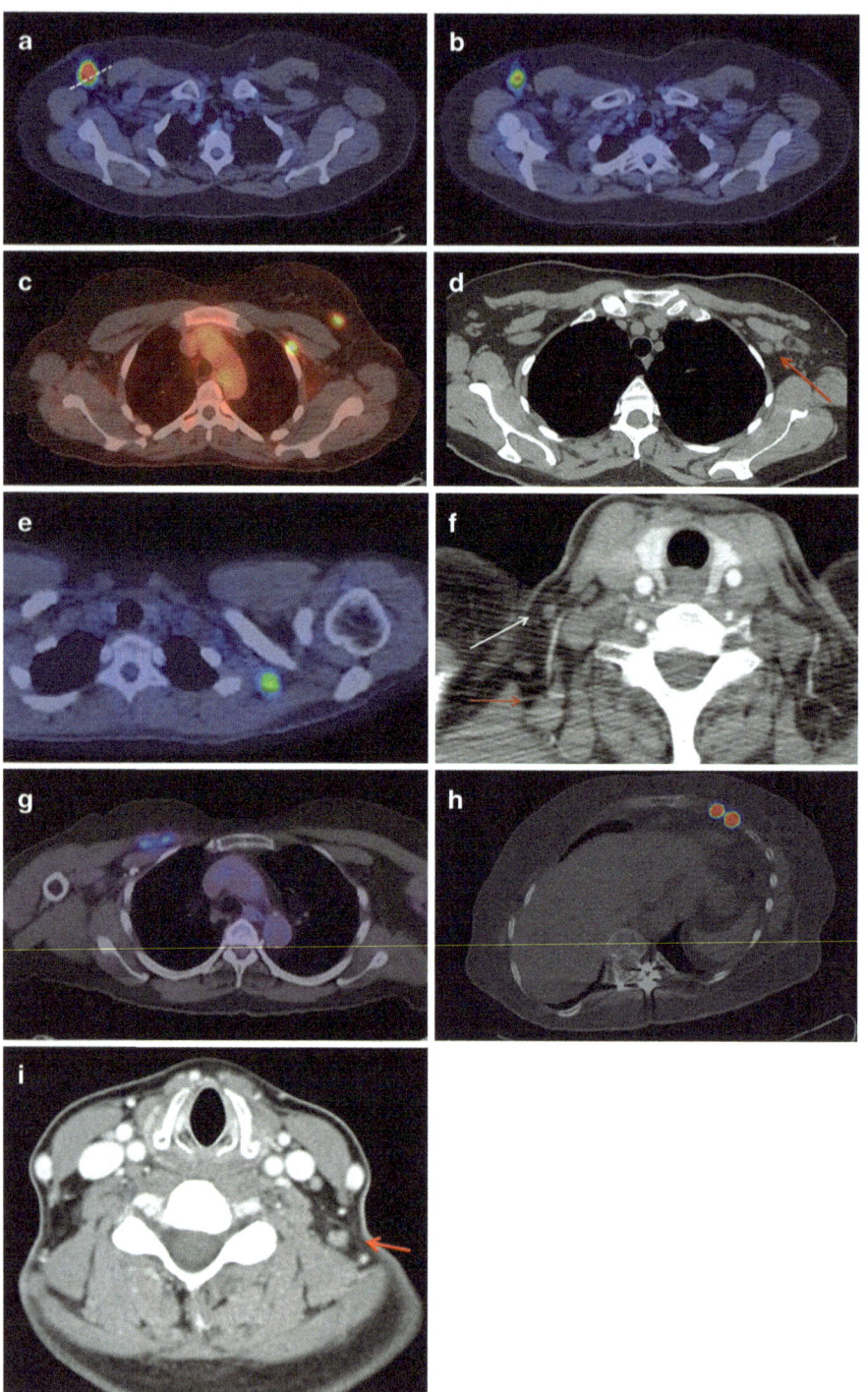

Gentile and colleagues mapped pre-neoadjuvant chemotherapy clinical lymph node involvement from diagnostic scans onto postoperative RT treatment planning scans of 30 patients with locally advanced breast cancer [30]. In 29 of 30 patients in this study, a portion of a clinically involved lymph node lay outside of the RTOG axillary consensus guideline CTV. Similar to Macdonald and colleagues, a common site for extension outside of the level 1 CTV was anterior, with 80% of patients having tumor extension in that direction (Fig. 4.1a). In addition, 83% of patients had tumor extension cranial to the RTOG level 1 CTV (Fig. 4.1b). A third common site of extension outside of the RTOG axillary consensus guideline border was in the caudal direction. Thirty-three percent, 80%, and 30% of lymph nodes extended outside of the caudal border of levels 1, 2, and 3, respectively (Fig. 4.1c, d). Patients in this study had bulky lymph node involvement. Therefore, the locations of nodal presentations may not reflect the risk for microscopic tumor extension in all patients. Nevertheless, both studies provide several lessons to help inform axillary target volumes.

First, in patients with indications for axillary RT, more generous target delineation anterior to level 1 than the plane defined by the anterior surface of the pectoralis major and latissimus dorsi muscles, as suggested by the RTOG consensus (Table 4.1), should be considered. In patients treated with 3D conformal photon RT treatment planning, much of this area will be within the tangential treatment fields regardless of how the CTV is defined. However, that is not the case with more conformal treatments including proton therapy, suggesting careful delineation in this area is important. In general, extension of the axillary level 1 CTV volume at least 1 cm anterior to the plane defined by the anterior surface of the pectoralis major and latissimus dorsi muscles but limited to 5 mm from the skin surface may be reasonable (Fig. 4.2e–k). This would ensure coverage of most lymph nodes in the

---

Fig. 4.1 Nodal sites of involvement with breast cancer. (**a**) The *white dashed line* depicts the anterior border of level 1 of the axilla in the RTOG atlas (plane defined by the anterior surface of the pectoralis major and latissimus dorsi muscles). A PET/CT scan demonstrates a hypermetabolic lymph node with its epicenter anterior to this border from a patient with recurrent breast cancer after axillary lymph node dissection. (**b**) PET/CT scan at the level of the humeral head from the same patient shows the recurrence is located in the high axillary level 1 lymph nodal region, above the cranial border defined in the RTOG atlas (axillary vessels crossing the lateral edge of the pectoralis minor muscle). (**c, d**) PET/CT scan in a patient with stage II breast cancer (**c**) and CT scan in a patient with stage III breast cancer (**d**) depicting metastatic lymphadenopathy posterior to the pectoralis minor muscle in level 2 (**c**) and posterior and medial to the pectoralis minor muscle in levels 2 (highlighted by the *red arrow*) and 3 more medially (**d**). The epicenter of each of these lymph nodes lies significantly caudal to the caudal borders of levels 2 (axillary vessels cross the lateral edge of the pectoralis minor) and 3 (axillary vessels cross the medial edge of the pectoralis minor) as defined in the RTOG atlas. (**e, f**) PET/CT (**e**) and CT (**f**) scans in two women presenting with stage III breast cancer demonstrating supraclavicular nodes in the lateral supraclavicular group (**e**) and posterior triangle (**f**) of the neck, as highlighted by the white and red arrows, posterolateral to the posterior (anterior aspect of the scalene muscle) and lateral (lateral edge of the sternocleidomastoid muscle) supraclavicular borders in the RTOG atlas. (**g**) PET/CT scan in a woman with stage II breast cancer showing hypermetabolic lymphadenopathy within the interpectoral space. (**h**) A deep chest wall presentation in the intercostal muscle is shown at the inferior aspect of the breast in a woman with prior breast-conserving surgery. (**i**) A biopsy-proven lymph node, highlighted by the red arrow), located at the level of the thyroid cartilage in a woman presenting with locoregionally advanced breast cancer

Table 4.1 Recommended modifications to RTOG breast cancer atlas consensus definitions

	Supraclavicular	Axilla level 1	Axilla level 2	Axilla level 3	Internal mammary
Recommended modifications to RTOG consensus definitions	Posteriorly and laterally more generous coverage to include the posterior triangle and lateral supraclavicular nodes (level 5) should be strongly considered, particularly in high-risk patients. Limiting the medial border of the supraclavicular CTV to the medial edge of the internal jugular vein may be appropriate in some lower-risk women. Cranially, more generous coverage may be considered in patients with multiple or high supraclavicular nodes	Anteriorly, more generous coverage than the plane defined by the pectoralis major and latissimus dorsi muscles should be considered. Cranially, more generous coverage may be considered, particularly in high-risk patients	Cranially, we recommend more generous coverage to the pectoralis minor muscle insertion on the coracoid. Caudally, we recommend more generous coverage to the obliteration of the fat space between the pectoralis major and minor muscles. We recommend including the interpectoral space in patients undergoing regional nodal irradiation	Caudally, we recommend more generous coverage to the obliteration of the fat space between the pectoralis major and minor muscles and the chest wall	We recommend medial and lateral expansions on the RTOG CTV of 4 mm. Cranially, when feasible, we recommend more generous coverage to the most caudal extent of the supraclavicular volume at the junction of the internal mammary vein with the brachiocephalic vein, particularly in patients with lymphadenopathy elsewhere in the IMN chain and other high-risk scenarios. More caudal extension than the third intercostal space may be considered in patients with lymphadenopathy elsewhere in the IMN chain when feasible

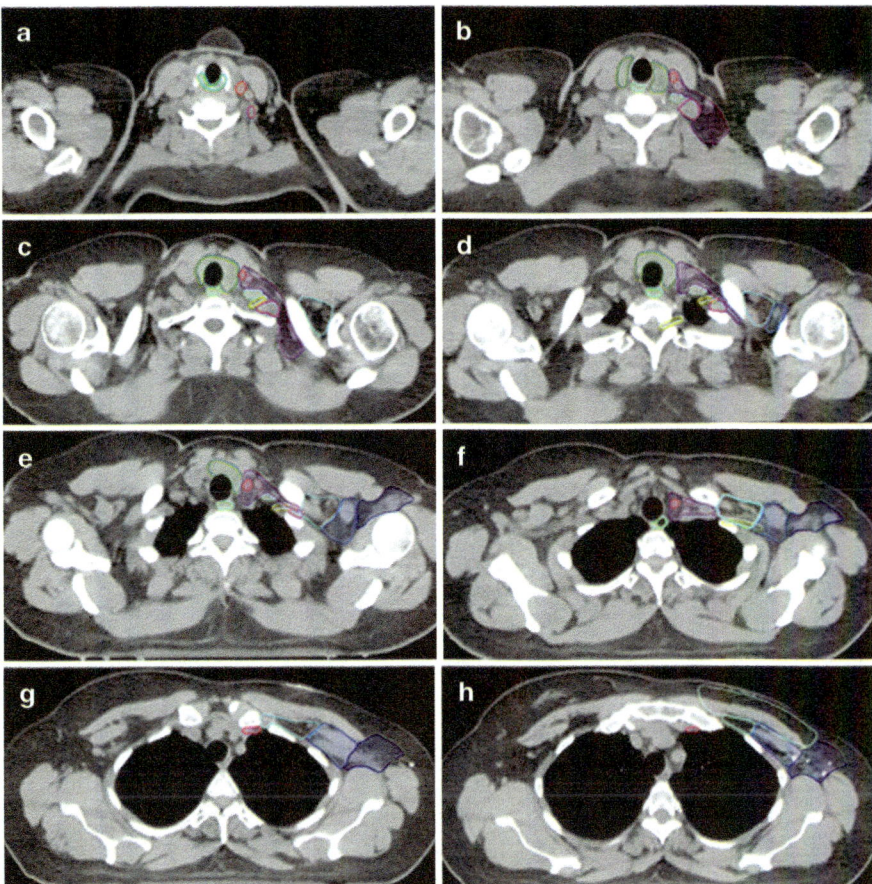

Fig. 4.2 (**a–p**) Representative axial slices with suggested CTV and normal tissue contours for postmastectomy radiotherapy are shown. (**q**) Sagittal view highlights the junction between the supraclavicular and internal mammary node (IMN) volumes, which are contiguously drawn (*red arrow*). This view also facilitates counting of the ribs to ensure the desired intercostal spaces are contoured. The cranial aspect of the fourth rib is shown by the *white arrow*. (**r**) Topogram view of the contours displays the CTV volumes as they relate to each other and the bony anatomy. The contiguous junction between the supraclavicular and IMN volume in this view is highlighted by the *orange arrow*. Physicians must weigh the risks of subclinical involvement in the most cranial extent of level 1 (*yellow arrow*) with the potential toxicity of treatment of this area when delineating the axillary CTV and may frequently reduce the cranial extent to minimize normal tissue exposure to the humeral head. In some high-risk patients, the axillary level 1 contour may extend slightly cranial to the most caudal extent of the humeral head, as drawn

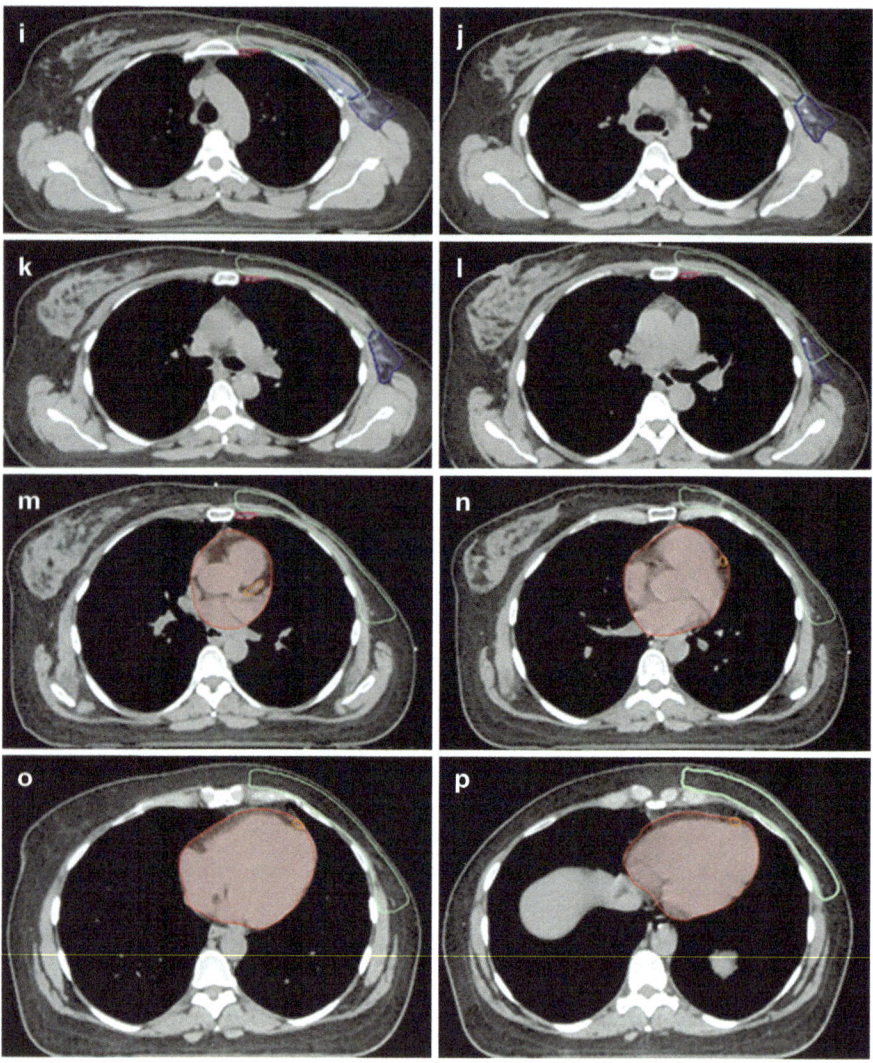

Fig. 4.2 (continued)

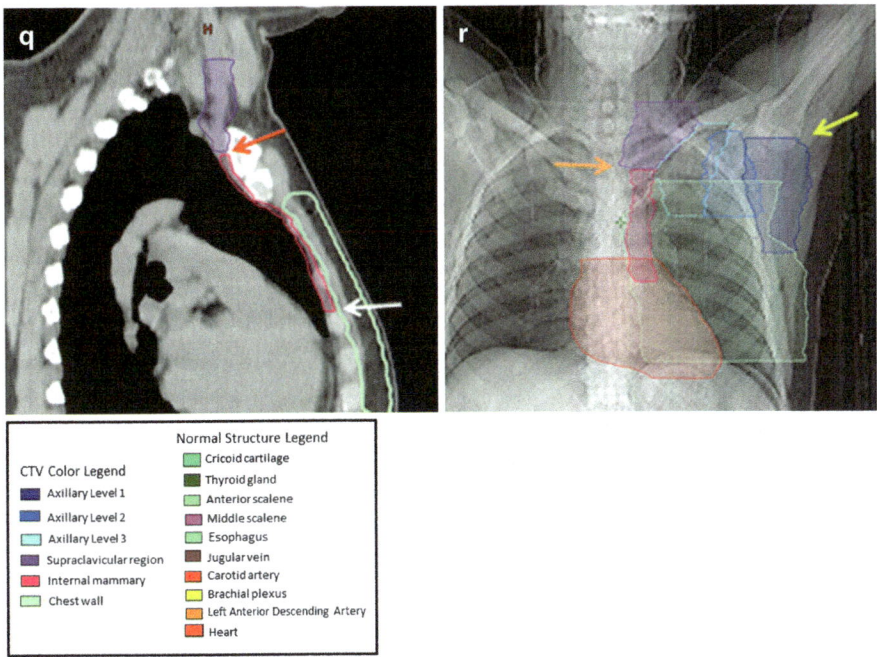

Fig. 4.2 (continued)

studies described above. Moreover, the work of Gentile and colleagues highlights the importance of careful review of pretherapy imaging during treatment planning in patients presenting with gross clinical lymphadenopathy to assist with target volume delineation here and elsewhere in the axilla. The location of postoperative changes such as seroma and axillary clips should be assessed to tailor the CTV for each individual patient to ensure regions at risk are adequately defined.

Second, the soft tissues in the axilla slightly above the cranial border of level 1 in the RTOG consensus (axillary vessels crossing the lateral edge of the pectoralis minor muscle) are at risk of harboring microscopic disease in many patients with indications for nodal irradiation (Fig. 4.1b). There is variation across atlases in terms of the recommended cranial border of axillary level 1 in Dijkema's anatomically based guidelines; the lateral axillary nodes extend superiorly along the latissimus dorsi tendon anterior to the humeral head [35], which is a notable difference between this and other atlases. By contrast, the Danish consensus atlas [12] defines the cranial margin of axillary level 1 as one cm below the humeral head. This less anatomically based definition is aligned with their historical target volumes, which they note have traditionally resulted in few local failures [12, 19]. With traditional 3D conformal treatment fields, the majority of level 1 is treated by the tangential fields whether they are specifically targeted or not. Targeting of the most cranial aspect of level 1, if desired, is accomplished by lateral extension of the supraclavicular field. More comprehensive targeting of the most cranial extent of level 1 has not been definitively associated with an increased risk of lymphedema [36] or improved disease control. Therefore, in delineating the axillary CTV in preparation for treatment planning with conventional 3D conformal breast cancer photon field arrangements, physicians must weigh the potential benefits of addressing residual microscopic disease in that location with the potential risks of increased tissue exposure of the humeral head and the draining lymphatics from the arm. Again, careful review of pretherapy imaging is important to ensure sites of initial gross clinical lymphadenopathy are addressed. In addition, consideration for more generous coverage of the most cranial aspect of level 1 may be reasonable in the setting of high axillary nodal burden, extranodal extension, inflammatory breast cancer, or poor response to neoadjuvant chemotherapy. Similarly, when the axilla is undissected, yet felt to be at high risk for microscopic disease, or in obese patients where the lymphatics may be less clearly defined, more generous coverage may be preferred. Alternatively, given the low rates of reported clinical failure, omission of this region for more favorable subsets undergoing regional nodal irradiation, such as those with low-volume disease identified elsewhere in the axilla who undergo a complete axillary lymph node dissection and those with a complete nodal response to chemotherapy, is unlikely to result in recurrence. Additionally, daily image guidance with attention to the humeral head may improve the accuracy of dose delivery and enable smaller PTV expansions into nontarget tissue.

Third, the axillary level 2 and 3 CTVs should be more generously contoured inferiorly than what is defined in the RTOG consensus, recognizing that in the context of traditional tangential photon treatment fields, this area will generally be treated regardless of the extent of the axillary CTV. In the study by Gentile and colleagues, 95% of lymph nodes were contained within 3.36 cm of the caudal level 2 border of the RTOG consensus and 2.21 cm of the caudal border of level 3 [30]. Therefore, in patients with indications for regional nodal irradiation, the axillary level 2 and 3 CTVs should extend caudally toward the insertion of the origin of the pectoralis minor muscle, transitioning into the breast and chest wall contours (discussed below) inferiorly (Fig. 4.2g–i).

More generally, controversy exists as to whether the dissected axilla should be routinely included in the CTV in patients with node-positive disease. Some have suggested that inclusion of levels 1 and 2 is unnecessary after axillary lymph node dissection [8]. They note that in the regional nodal irradiation arm of the National Cancer Institute of Canada MA.20 trial, few axillary failures were observed despite only approximately one third of patients with <10 axillary nodes removed or >3 positive nodes having all three levels of the axilla comprehensively treated by extending the lateral border of the supraclavicular field to encompass the surgical neck of the humerus [2]. For approximately two thirds of women treated with ≥10 axillary nodes removed and ≤3 nodes positive, the MA.20 protocol defined that the supraclavicular field extend laterally to the medial edge of the humeral head but include the coracoid process. Consequently, if treated according to protocol, a small portion of the axilla lateral to that border, but above the match line with the tangential fields, was not intentionally targeted in those patients. However, it is noteworthy that even with that less comprehensive supraclavicular field design, most of axillary levels 1 and 2 receives a therapeutic dose from the tangential fields and the lateral portion of the supraclavicular field, regardless of whether they are intentionally targeted [37]. Similarly, nodal radiation is only to be directed to the "undissected axilla" in patients randomized to the axillary lymph node dissection arm of Alliance 11202, A Randomized Phase III Trial Comparing Axillary Lymph Node Dissection to Axillary Radiation in Breast Cancer Patients (cT1-3N1) Who Have Positive Sentinel Lymph Node Disease After Neoadjuvant Chemotherapy, whereas the full axilla is targeted in the sentinel lymph node biopsy only arm (NCT01901094). However, as in MA.20, a large majority of the axilla will be encompassed with traditional photon tangential fields below the match line and the lateral portion of the supraclavicular field in both arms. In contrast, in patients treated with conformal techniques like proton therapy, much of the dissected axilla can truly be avoided when treating the breast or chest wall if desired. Therefore, physicians should be cautious when extrapolating the results of clinical trials addressing the management of the axilla in patients treated with photon radiotherapy as they delineate the CTV. In women with indications for regional nodal irradiation who are treated with proton therapy, our current practice is to include levels 1 and 2 of the axilla in the CTV, irrespective of whether an axillary lymph node dissection was performed [25, 37]. Further research will be needed to determine the most appropriate extent of the axillary CTV in this setting. The results of Alliance 11202 and NSABP B51, A Randomized Phase III Clinical Trial Evaluating Post-Mastectomy Chestwall and Regional Nodal XRT and Post-Lumpectomy Regional Nodal XRT in Patients with Positive Axillary Nodes Before Neoadjuvant Chemotherapy Who Convert to Pathologically Negative Axillary Nodes After Neoadjuvant Chemotherapy (NCT01872975) will help inform the optimal management of the axilla in the years ahead.

4.3   Supraclavicular Volume

One accessory route of lymphatic vessels originating in the upper part of the breast is to follow the cutaneous branches of the thoracoacromial artery, with some vessels potentially extending to the supraclavicular lymph nodes [32]. In patients with node-positive breast cancer treated with mastectomy and chemotherapy without nodal irradiation, the supraclavicular region is at risk of locoregional recurrence [38, 39]. Key anatomic structures used to define the supraclavicular region are the trapezius, platysma, sternocleidomastoid, levator scapulae, and scalene muscles along with the cricoid cartilage, common carotid artery, and internal jugular vein [40]. Historically, a classic supraclavicular field was directed from an anterior-oblique direction at an angle of approximately 12–15°. The medial border of this field was at midline and a medial block was drawn using the transverse processes of the cervical spine or a wire over the anterior edge of the sternocleidomastoid muscle as landmarks to spare midline structures including the esophagus, thyroid, and spinal cord [12, 41]. The supraclavicular field was matched to the tangential fields near the inferior portion of the clavicular head, while the superior border flashed the shoulder [41]. Standard photon supraclavicular field targets have been compared with sites of supraclavicular lymph node positivity by PET scan, identifying the medial border of the field and the region posterior to the vertebral body transverse process as potential sites of geographic miss [41]. Standard fields based solely on bony landmarks with uniform prescription depths should no longer be used in the 3D era of CTV-based planning due to the potential for suboptimal target coverage [9, 10].

Recently, the position of involved supraclavicular nodes at presentation and at recurrence relative to consensus guideline CTV contours has been examined, providing guidance for the generation of the supraclavicular CTV for modern RT planning [31, 42]. Brown and colleagues from the Mayo Clinic identified 62 patients with 161 supraclavicular nodal metastases. The locations of the nodes were transferred onto representative axial CT images and compared with the supraclavicular CTV generated using the RTOG breast cancer atlas which closely resembles levels 4a and 5b of the head and neck consensus guidelines published by Grégoire and colleagues encompassing the lower jugular and medial supraclavicular nodes [40]. Of the 161 nodal metastases, 39 % were outside of the RTOG volume. Two of the most common locations for lymph nodes outside of the RTOG volume were in the posterior triangle (posterolateral to the RTOG volume) and in the lateral supraclavicular group (lateral to the RTOG volume), including isolated nodal failures in these regions (Fig. 4.1e, f) [42]. These areas correspond to level 5 and 5c in the updated head and neck consensus [40]. Another common location of supraclavicular disease outside of the RTOG volume was superiorly, in the vicinity of the cricoid and thyroid cartilage (Fig. 4.1i). However, all women with nodal disease in that location had multiple supraclavicular metastases, suggesting that extension of volumes into this area may be a consideration in patients with more advanced regional presentations of the disease.

Jing and colleagues from China performed a similar analysis, mapping the location of metastatic supraclavicular lymph nodes in 55 patients. Locations of nodes were compared to supraclavicular CTVs from a variety of atlases, including the atlas from RTOG [31]. Strikingly similar findings to the previously reported study were observed, with 38 % of lymph nodes falling outside of the RTOG CTV. Again, an important location of lymphadenopathy outside of the RTOG CTV was in the posterolateral direction in the posterior triangle and lateral supraclavicular regions. In addition, Jing et al. identified the junction of the jugular and subclavian veins as a common location of lymphadenopathy with 66 % of patients having nodes within 5 mm of the confluence of these vessels (Fig. 4.2q, r).

These studies highlight several important points that should be considered in the management of patients with indications for supraclavicular RT. First, the available evidence suggests that lymph nodes in the posterior triangle and lateral supraclavicular region of the neck below the cricoid cartilage are targets for the majority of women undergoing regional nodal irradiation for breast cancer [26, 31, 41, 42]. Although a high number of lymph nodes in these locations were outside of the RTOG defined CTV, that does not imply that these areas are inadequately treated in traditional fields designed to target the RTOG CTV. Indeed, with an anterior-oblique supraclavicular field designed to deliver the prescription dose to the RTOG supraclavicular CTV, most of the lymph nodes in the posterior triangle and lateral supraclavicular regions will generally receive at least 90 % of the prescription dose [26]. Therefore, these areas are treated in the CTV-based breast planning era, just as they were with historical bony landmark-based fields [26, 41]. By the same rationale, including this more posterolateral nodal region in the CTV is unlikely to result in greater toxicity in patients treated with 3D conformal photon treatment, as some have suggested. In contrast, for patients treated with proton therapy, targeting only the RTOG supraclavicular CTV would result in minimal exposure to the posterior triangle and lateral supraclavicular nodal region areas and be a deintensification of treatment. Therefore, outside of a protocol, when using proton therapy, we recommend more generous coverage of the supraclavicular fossa, as has been proposed by others [28, 42].

Second, the optimal superior extent of the CTV for elective nodal irradiation of the supraclavicular lymph nodes remains an area of controversy. Based on cadaver dissection and radiology study, one group proposed that the superior border should begin at the level of the thyrocricoid membrane [10]. Others, based on expert consensus, proposed the cranial edge of the subclavian arch as the cranial border [14, 43], underscoring the variability that exists even among experts. Given the available evidence and low rates of nodal failure above the cricoid cartilage, we recommend that the supraclavicular volume generally begin at the inferior border of the cricoid cartilage. However, in the setting of multiple supraclavicular metastases or a superiorly located supraclavicular metastasis in the vicinity of the cricoid cartilage, we recommend extending the border of the volume cranially to at least the thyroid cartilage [26].

Third, lymphadenopathy medial to the internal carotid artery is extremely unusual. Therefore, the anterior jugular, paratracheal, pretracheal, and prelaryngeal lymph nodes (level 6 of the neck, as defined by Grégoire and colleagues) are not targets in women undergoing elective nodal RT for breast cancer, and the elective CTV should not abut the esophagus [28]. The location of the medial border may be particularly relevant in left-sided patients where the esophagus may approximate the common carotid artery. In addition, in patients treated with proton therapy ranging out into the esophagus may occur, depending on the beam angles and margins used with planning. In the absence of gross disease in the vicinity of the carotid sheath, the supraclavicular CTV should extend no further medially than the medial border of the common carotid artery (Fig. 4.2a–f). Physicians must carefully balance the potential risks of esophagitis [28] and secondary esophageal malignancy with coverage in this area [6]. In some women with indications for elective regional nodal irradiation but low risk of supraclavicular recurrence, even less comprehensive coverage may be pursued here, as some atlases suggest. For example, low rates of regional failure have previously been reported in early-stage breast cancer when the medial supraclavicular field edge border was placed at the anterior edge of the sternocleidomastoid muscle, and lymphadenopathy near the carotid artery was unusual in the supraclavicular mapping studies of Brown et al. and Jing et al. [31, 42]. Limiting the medial border of the supraclavicular CTV at the internal jugular vein may be a reasonable approach to CTV-based planning in some lower-risk women [12, 14, 43]. The use of image guidance to minimize the planning target volume expansion and day-to-day setup uncertainty may be considered [44].

4.4   Interpectoral Nodes

While not separately noted as a separate target volume within some of the available atlases, the interpectoral or Rotter's nodes are a region at risk for lymph node involvement (Fig. 4.1g). Lymphatic channels pass throw the fascicles of the pectoralis major, where some are interrupted by the interpectoral nodes and others proceed to the apical axilla or clavicular nodes [32]. This volume is included in our recommended nodal and chest wall CTV and should be included when other nodal volumes are targeted.

4.5   Breast/Chest Wall Contouring Guidelines

The target volume for the breast generally includes all visible glandular breast tissue. That said, in most patients undergoing whole breast radiotherapy for DCIS and early invasive breast cancer, the far most medial and lateral extent of the breast tissue many centimeters away from the lumpectomy cavity is at no higher risk of recurrence than the contralateral breast [45–47]. The lumpectomy cavity should be contoured in all patients to identify the area at highest risk of recurrence. In many situations minimizing exposure to the organs at risk may take precedence over delivering 100 % of prescription to all visible glandular breast tissue on imaging distant from the lumpectomy cavity. For example, it would be extremely unusual for a patient undergoing whole breast irradiation in our practice to have a mean heart dose >1 Gy. Identification of the breast tissue on CT scan may be facilitated by the placement of radiopaque wires at the time of simulation, marking the clinical borders of the breast mound. Due to the buildup region at the body surface, by convention for the purposes of dose reporting, the breast CTV is generally inclusive of the glandular tissue, up to 5 mm beneath the surface of the skin, except in particular circumstances where full dose to the skin is required. Our recommended breast CTV does not include the pectoralis muscles, except when nodal radiation is indicated. In the latter setting, perforating lymphatic pathways pass through the pectoralis muscles [32] and are at risk for subclinical involvement.

Inclusion of the ribs and intercostal muscles to the pleura within the postmastectomy chest wall CTV varies within consensus guidelines [12, 15, 43]. This area has historically been treated due to the geometry of traditional photon tangential beams. A recent report reviewed published postmastectomy recurrences [29]. The majority (72–100 %) occurred within the skin and subcutaneous tissue, with an additional 25 % within the pectoralis muscles, and there were no reported isolated recurrence in the intercostal muscle or ribs [29]. Another detailed study identified 28 % of recurrences deep to the skin or subcutaneous tissue and importantly highlighted the potential bias in identifying more superficially located recurrences [48]. Given that a notable portion of recurrences are within the pectoralis muscles (Fig. 4.1g), and the known lymphatic pathways through this region [32], it is our general practice to include these structures in the chest wall CTV definition in patients undergoing PMRT. Even deeper recurrences are reported [49, 50] (Fig. 4.1h) but seem to be associated with more advanced, full-thickness presentation, suggesting that there is low likelihood of first recurrence at the ribs or intercostal muscles for most women. Based on the perceived lower risk to the deeper tissues, we recommend the CTV extend up to but not include the ribs and intercostal muscles for the majority of PMRT and postlumpectomy patients with indications for regional nodal irradiation. Limiting the CTV in this way may significantly reduce dose to the heart and lung in some patients, particularly those treated with electrons, IMRT, or proton therapy. Consideration for deeper coverage to include the intercostal muscles or ribs may be appropriate in advanced settings where data are limited and the risk of recurrence is higher, such as inflammatory breast cancer, extensive lymphovascular invasion, direct chest wall invasion, or clinical internal mammary involvement. As in all sites, an appropriate PTV expansion based on the setup and treatment uncertainties specific to each institution should be added.

4.6   Internal Mammary Nodes (IMNs)

An alternative lymphatic drainage pathway from the breast is along the cutaneous perforating branches of the internal thoracic (internal mammary) artery and vein. These lymphatics perforate the pectoralis major and intercostal muscles, draining into the IMNs [32]. Although clinically detected isolated recurrences in the IMNs are unusual, recent prospective clinical data suggests that clinically undetected disease in the IMNs may be a relatively important source of distant spread in women with node-positive breast cancer [2, 3, 23]. Similar to the other nodal regions, there are discrepancies in CTV recommendations between the various consensus volumes and atlases.

Radical mastectomy studies and autopsy series have demonstrated that the highest-risk region for IMNs is the first three intercostal spaces. Lymphoscintigraphy of clinical stage I and II breast patients demonstrates very few nodes at the fourth intercostal space or beyond [51, 52]. Similarly, in a series of 112 RT patients with radiographic evidence of internal mammary nodal involvement, the location was within the first three intercostal spaces in all but one case [53]. Consistent with these studies, the ESTRO and RTOG guidelines suggest the cranial aspect of the fourth rib [43], whereas the Danish Cooperative group recommends the superior aspect of the fifth rib as the caudal border [12]. Our own unpublished data suggests that IMN involvement caudal to the third intercostal space is unusual in the absence of gross IMN lymphadenopathy in the first three intercostal spaces (under review). Therefore, our general recommendation is to include the first three intercostal spaces for elective IMN coverage. Rarely, this may be extended where risk is deemed to be higher, such as in the setting of known clinical internal mammary node involvement. Similarly, for locally advanced primary tumors along the lower-inner breast, slightly more generous coverage may also be considered.

The superior border of the RTOG and Danish atlases are at the superior aspect of the medial first rib. However, the space surrounding the junction of the jugular, subclavian, and internal mammary veins has been reported to be associated with a relatively high rate of nodal involvement [31]. Therefore, similar to other published guidelines, we recommend that the cranial aspect of the IMN volume meet the supraclavicular nodes whenever possible (Fig. 4.2q, r) [12, 15, 35, 43]. This is accomplished by following the internal mammary vein back to the point where it empties (along with the subclavian and internal jugular veins), into the brachiocephalic vein. Depending on the technique employed, comprehensive coverage of the IMNs at their most cranial extent immediately below the match line is technically challenging with photons or electrons due to the depth of the IMNs at this location (Fig. 4.2g, h) and may result in significantly more normal tissue exposure. As a result, some have recommended exclusion of this junction in the CTV [12]. We recommend careful review of individual patient anatomy and plan evaluation, with consideration of omission of coverage when recurrence risk is felt to be low, and targeting this juncture will markedly increase normal tissue exposure. In the setting of proton therapy, this juncture of the IMN and supraclavicular CTV can be treated with relatively minimal additional dose to organs at risk. Therefore, we routinely include this area in patients with indications for regional nodal irradiation who are treated with proton therapy. Finally, the optimal extent of the medial and lateral borders for the IMN CTV is an area of uncertainty. The RTOG atlas limits the internal mammary node CTV to inclusion of the internal mammary vessels, whereas others have suggested a 5 mm margin on the internal mammary vein, or internal mammary vessels may be appropriate [12, 35, 43]. We recently mapped the location of 115 gross IMN metastases relative to the internal mammary vessels in order to guide the delineation of the IMN CTV (Mutter et al. under review). Ninety percent of lymph nodes would be encompassed with a 4 mm expansion on the internal mammary vessels medially and laterally. Posteriorly, we do not recommend extending the IMN CTV into the lung; however, an institutionally appropriate PTV which also accounts for respiratory motion may be added.

4.7   Organs at Risk

Contouring for breast cancer should include organs at risk, with doses to these structures considered as part of plan evaluation. We recommend routine contouring of the bilateral lung, heart, spinal cord, esophagus, and ipsilateral brachial plexus, particularly when boost doses to adjacent nodal regions are planned. Contouring and limiting dose to the left anterior descending and right coronary arteries in patients undergoing left-sided and right-sided radiotherapy, respectively, is also appropriate given concern regarding the potential risk of late cardiac toxicity with even low doses of radiotherapy [7]. Attention should also be paid to the humeral head and joint space, the trachea, the thyroid, and the contralateral breast. In women treated with multibeam intensity-modulated therapy, there is also potential for low-dose spread to nontarget organs and tissues. Therefore, in such cases, clinicians must also be cognizant of dose to the esophagus, liver (for right-sided cases), and stomach (for left-sided cases). For delineation of the cardiac structures, the University of Michigan has published a cardiac atlas with detailed guidelines [54]. Similarly, reference atlases for the delineation of the brachial plexus may guide contouring [55, 56].

Conclusion

Advances in systemic therapy and other aspects of the breast cancer multidisciplinary practice have lead to a reduction in recurrence risk over time. These improvements, combined with a greater appreciation for the potential late effects of ionizing radiation, have resulted in coordinated efforts to de-intensify breast cancer RT in appropriately selected patients. For example, clinical trials are under way to determine whether RT may be safely omitted in women with node-positive breast cancer with excellent responses to preoperative chemotherapy. Genomic classifiers are also rapidly being incorporated into practice, with promise to identify patients at low risk of recurrence, helping identify which patients are unlikely to benefit from treatment. At the same time, our understanding of the potential benefits of carefully directed RT in subsets of patients has expanded. Studies of regional nodal treatment have demonstrated that sterilizing subclinical locoregional disease results in a greater reduction in distant metastases than locoregional recurrence, implying that a clinically undetected locoregional disease is a more frequent source of distant relapse than originally thought [2, 3]. The rapid incorporation of technology into the clinic has revolutionized the RT practice, providing greater opportunity to deliver RT to the target more accurately than ever before, without exposing normal tissues. Therefore, as areas at risk of harboring microscopic disease in the modern era are better understood and target volumes further refined, there is a real opportunity to improve the therapeutic ratio in the years ahead. In order to maximize this opportunity, more study will be required to better understand patterns of relapse in patients with varying clinical characteristics and tumor biology. This will enable an era of "precision" breast cancer radiotherapy where RT targets are truly personalized to the risk profile of each individual patient, and normal tissue exposure is reduced with technological advances in RT delivery.

References

1. Darby S, McGale P, Correa C et al (2011) Effect of radiotherapy after breast-conserving surgery on 10-year recurrence and 15-year breast cancer death: meta-analysis of individual patient data for 10,801 women in 17 randomised trials. Lancet 378:1707–1716
2. Whelan TJ, Olivotto IA, Parulekar WR et al (2015) Regional nodal irradiation in early-stage breast cancer. N Engl J Med 373:307–316
3. Poortmans PM, Collette S, Kirkove C et al (2015) Internal mammary and medial supraclavicular irradiation in breast cancer. N Engl J Med 373:317–327
4. McGale P, Taylor C, Correa C et al (2014) Effect of radiotherapy after mastectomy and axillary surgery on 10-year recurrence and 20-year breast cancer mortality: meta-analysis of individual patient data for 8135 women in 22 randomised trials. Lancet 383:2127–2135

5. Warren LE, Miller CL, Horick N et al (2014) The impact of radiation therapy on the risk of lymphedema after treatment for breast cancer: a prospective cohort study. Int J Radiat Oncol Biol Phys 88:565–571
6. Clarke M, Collins R, Darby S et al (2005) Effects of radiotherapy and of differences in the extent of surgery for early breast cancer on local recurrence and 15-year survival: an overview of the randomised trials. Lancet 366:2087–2106
7. Darby SC, Ewertz M, McGale P et al (2013) Risk of ischemic heart disease in women after radiotherapy for breast cancer. N Engl J Med 368:987–998
8. White J (2015) Defining target volumes in breast cancer radiation therapy for the future: back to basics. Int J Radiat Oncol Biol Phys 93:277–280
9. Bentel GC, Marks LB, Hardenbergh PH, Prosnitz LR (2000) Variability of the depth of supra-clavicular and axillary lymph nodes in patients with breast cancer: is a posterior axillary boost field necessary? Int J Radiat Oncol Biol Phys 47:755–758
10. Madu CN, Quint DJ, Normolle DP, Marsh RB, Wang EY, Pierce LJ (2001) Definition of the supraclavicular and infraclavicular nodes: implications for three-dimensional CT-based conformal radiation therapy. Radiology 221:333–339
11. Munshi A, Mallick I, Budrukkar A et al (2008) A novel method for CT-scan-based localization of the internal mammary chain by internal mammary catheterization: an aid in breast cancer radiation therapy planning. Br J Radiol 81:485–489
12. Nielsen MH, Berg M, Pedersen AN et al (2013) Delineation of target volumes and organs at risk in adjuvant radiotherapy of early breast cancer: national guidelines and contouring atlas by the Danish Breast Cancer Cooperative Group. Acta Oncol 52:703–710
13. Atean I, Pointreau Y, Ouldamer L et al (2013) A simplified CT-based definition of the supraclavicular and infraclavicular nodal volumes in breast cancer. Cancer Radiother 17:39–43
14. Verhoeven K, Weltens C, Remouchamps V et al (2015) Vessel based delineation guidelines for the elective lymph node regions in breast cancer radiation therapy – PROCAB guidelines. Radiother Oncol 114:11–16
15. Breast cancer atlas for radiation therapy planning: consensus definition (Accessed 15 Feb 2016, at https://www.rtog.org/LinkClick.aspx?fileticket=vzJFhPaBipE%3d&tabid=236)
16. Hurkmans CW, Borger JH, Pieters BR, Russell NS, Jansen EP, Mijnheer BJ (2001) Variability in target volume delineation on CT scans of the breast. Int J Radiat Oncol Biol Phys 50:1366–1372
17. Li XA, Tai A, Arthur DW et al (2009) Variability of target and normal structure delineation for breast cancer radiotherapy: an RTOG Multi-Institutional and Multiobserver Study. Int J Radiat Oncol Biol Phys 73:944–951
18. Struikmans H, Warlam-Rodenhuis C, Stam T et al (2005) Interobserver variability of clinical target volume delineation of glandular breast tissue and of boost volume in tangential breast irradiation. Radiother Oncol 76:293–299
19. Nielsen HM, Offersen BV (2015) Regional recurrence after adjuvant breast cancer radiotherapy is not due to insufficient target coverage. Radiother Oncol 114:1–2
20. Thorsen LB, Thomsen MS, Berg M et al (2014) CT-planned internal mammary node radiotherapy in the DBCG-IMN study: benefit versus potentially harmful effects. Acta Oncol 53:1027–1034
21. Fontanilla HP, Woodward WA, Lindberg ME et al (2012) Current clinical coverage of Radiation Therapy Oncology Group-defined target volumes for postmastectomy radiation therapy. Pract Radiat Oncol 2:201–209
22. Macdonald SM, Patel SA, Hickey S et al (2013) Proton therapy for breast cancer after mastectomy: early outcomes of a prospective clinical trial. Int J Radiat Oncol Biol Phys 86:484–490
23. Thorsen LB, Offersen BV, Dano H et al (2016) DBCG-IMN: a population-based cohort study on the effect of internal mammary node irradiation in early node-positive breast cancer. J Clin Oncol 34:314–320
24. MacDonald SM, Jimenez R, Paetzold P et al (2013) Proton radiotherapy for chest wall and regional lymphatic radiation; dose comparisons and treatment delivery. Radiat Oncol 8:71

25. Giuliano AE, Hunt KK, Ballman KV et al (2011) Axillary dissection vs no axillary dissection in women with invasive breast cancer and sentinel node metastasis: a randomized clinical trial. JAMA 305:569–575
26. Brown LC, Diehn FE, Boughey JC et al (2015) Delineation of supraclavicular target volumes in breast cancer radiation therapy. In reply to Yang and Guo. Int J Radiat Oncol Biol Phys 93:723–724
27. Jagsi R, Chadha M, Moni J et al (2014) Radiation field design in the ACOSOG Z0011 (Alliance) Trial. J Clin Oncol 32:3600–3606
28. Cuaron JJ, Chon B, Tsai H et al (2015) Early toxicity in patients treated with postoperative proton therapy for locally advanced breast cancer. Int J Radiat Oncol Biol Phys 92: 284–291
29. Vargo JA, Beriwal S (2015) RTOG chest wall contouring guidelines for post-mastectomy radiation therapy: is It evidence-based? Int J Radiat Oncol Biol Phys 93:266–267
30. Gentile MS, Usman AA, Neuschler EI, Sathiaseelan V, Hayes JP, Small W Jr (2015) Contouring guidelines for the axillary lymph nodes for the delivery of radiation therapy in breast cancer: evaluation of the RTOG breast cancer atlas. Int J Radiat Oncol Biol Phys 93:257–265
31. Jing H, Wang SL, Li J et al (2015) Mapping patterns of ipsilateral supraclavicular nodal metastases in breast cancer: rethinking the clinical target volume for high-risk patients. Int J Radiat Oncol Biol Phys 93:268–276
32. Lengele B, Nyssen-Behets C, Scalliet P (2007) Anatomical bases for the radiological delineation of lymph node areas. Upper limbs, chest and abdomen. Radiother Oncol 84:335–347
33. Donker M, van Tienhoven G, Straver ME et al (2014) Radiotherapy or surgery of the axilla after a positive sentinel node in breast cancer (EORTC 10981–22023 AMAROS): a randomised, multicentre, open-label, phase 3 non-inferiority trial. Lancet Oncol 15:1303–1310
34. MacDonald SM, Harisinghani MG, Katkar A, Napolitano B, Wolfgang J, Taghian AG (2010) Nanoparticle-enhanced MRI to evaluate radiation delivery to the regional lymphatics for patients with breast cancer. Int J Radiat Oncol Biol Phys 77:1098–1104
35. Dijkema IM, Hofman P, Raaijmakers CP, Lagendijk JJ, Battermann JJ, Hillen B (2004) Locoregional conformal radiotherapy of the breast: delineation of the regional lymph node clinical target volumes in treatment position. Radiother Oncol 71:287–295
36. Chandra RA, Miller CL, Skolny MN et al (2015) Radiation therapy risk factors for development of lymphedema in patients treated with regional lymph node irradiation for breast cancer. Int J Radiat Oncol Biol Phys 91:760–764
37. Schlembach PJ, Buchholz TA, Ross MI et al (2001) Relationship of sentinel and axillary level I-II lymph nodes to tangential fields used in breast irradiation. Int J Radiat Oncol Biol Phys 51:671–678
38. Recht A, Gray R, Davidson NE et al (1999) Locoregional failure 10 years after mastectomy and adjuvant chemotherapy with or without tamoxifen without irradiation: experience of the Eastern Cooperative Oncology Group. J Clin Oncol 17:1689–1700
39. Katz A, Strom EA, Buchholz TA et al (2000) Locoregional recurrence patterns after mastectomy and doxorubicin-based chemotherapy: implications for postoperative irradiation. J Clin Oncol 18:2817–2827
40. Gregoire V, Ang K, Budach W et al (2014) Delineation of the neck node levels for head and neck tumors: a 2013 update. DAHANCA, EORTC, HKNPCSG, NCIC CTG, NCRI, RTOG, TROG consensus guidelines. Radiother Oncol 110:172–181
41. Reed VK, Cavalcanti JL, Strom EA et al (2008) Risk of subclinical micrometastatic disease in the supraclavicular nodal bed according to the anatomic distribution in patients with advanced breast cancer. Int J Radiat Oncol Biol Phys 71:435–440
42. Brown LC, Diehn FE, Boughey JC et al (2015) Delineation of supraclavicular target volumes in breast cancer radiation therapy. Int J Radiat Oncol Biol Phys 92:642–649
43. Offersen BV, Boersma LJ, Kirkove C et al (2015) ESTRO consensus guideline on target volume delineation for elective radiation therapy of early stage breast cancer. Radiother Oncol 114:3–10

44. Dawson LA, Sharpe MB (2006) Image-guided radiotherapy: rationale, benefits, and limitations. Lancet Oncol 7:848–858
45. Smith TE, Lee D, Turner BC, Carter D, Haffty BG (2000) True recurrence vs. new primary ipsilateral breast tumor relapse: an analysis of clinical and pathologic differences and their implications in natural history, prognoses, and therapeutic management. Int J Radiat Oncol Biol Phys 48:1281–1289
46. Huang E, Buchholz TA, Meric F et al (2002) Classifying local disease recurrences after breast conservation therapy based on location and histology: new primary tumors have more favorable outcomes than true local disease recurrences. Cancer 95:2059–2067
47. Strnad V, Ott OJ, Hildebrandt G et al (2016) 5-year results of accelerated partial breast irradiation using sole interstitial multicatheter brachytherapy versus whole-breast irradiation with boost after breast-conserving surgery for low-risk invasive and in-situ carcinoma of the female breast: a randomised, phase 3, non-inferiority trial. Lancet 387:229–238
48. Langstein HN, Cheng MH, Singletary SE et al (2003) Breast cancer recurrence after immediate reconstruction: patterns and significance. Plast Reconstr Surg 111:712–720; discussion 21–22
49. Levy Faber D, Fadel E, Kolb F et al (2013) Outcome of full-thickness chest wall resection for isolated breast cancer recurrence. Eur J Cardiothorac Surg 44:637–642
50. Friedel G, Kuipers T, Engel C et al (2005) Full-thickness chest wall resection for locally recurrent breast cancer. Thorac Surg Sci 2:Doc01
51. Recht A, Siddon RL, Kaplan WD, Andersen JW, Harris JR (1988) Three-dimensional internal mammary lymphoscintigraphy: implications for radiation therapy treatment planning for breast carcinoma. Int J Radiat Oncol Biol Phys 14:477–481
52. Kaplan WD, Andersen JW, Siddon RL et al (1988) The three-dimensional localization of internal mammary lymph nodes by radionuclide lymphoscintigraphy. J Nucl Med 29:473–478
53. Zhang YJ, Oh JL, Whitman GJ et al (2010) Clinically apparent internal mammary nodal metastasis in patients with advanced breast cancer: incidence and local control. Int J Radiat Oncol Biol Phys 77:1113–1119
54. Feng M, Moran JM, Koelling T et al (2011) Development and validation of a heart atlas to study cardiac exposure to radiation following treatment for breast cancer. Int J Radiat Oncol Biol Phys 79:10–18
55. Truong MT, Nadgir RN, Hirsch AE et al (2010) Brachial plexus contouring with CT and MR imaging in radiation therapy planning for head and neck cancer. Radiographics 30:1095–1103
56. Hall WH, Guiou M, Lee NY et al (2008) Development and validation of a standardized method for contouring the brachial plexus: preliminary dosimetric analysis among patients treated with IMRT for head-and-neck cancer. Int J Radiat Oncol Biol Phys 72:1362–1367

Accelerated Partial Breast Irradiation (APBI)

5

Rachel B. Jimenez

Contents

5.1 Overview

Among women with early-stage breast cancer who undergo breast-conserving surgery, adjuvant whole breast radiation has traditionally been the standard of care. Over the past 20 years however, accelerated partial breast irradiation (APBI) has gained increasing attention as an alternative for select patients by delivering adjuvant radiation therapy to a limited region of the breast at highest risk of recurrence. This approach minimizes the amount of normal tissue receiving radiation, e.g., the lung, heart, and chest wall, while also enabling delivery of a higher dose per fraction

R.B. Jimenez, MD (✉)
Department of Radiation Oncology, Massachusetts General Hospital, Boston, MA, USA
e-mail: rbjimenez@partners.org

© Springer International Publishing Switzerland 2016
J.R. Bellon et al. (eds.), *Radiation Therapy Techniques and Treatment Planning for Breast Cancer*, Practical Guides in Radiation Oncology,
DOI 10.1007/978-3-319-40392-2_5

61

to confer an overall shorter treatment duration compared to whole breast radiation therapy (WBRT).

The rationale for APBI comes from the results of multiple randomized trials comparing mastectomy to breast-conserving surgery with or without adjuvant whole breast radiation [1, 2]. In these studies, the majority of ipsilateral breast recurrences were located in proximity to the lumpectomy cavity, suggesting that a more conformal radiation treatment might equally mitigate the risk of local recurrence. In the intervening years, techniques used to deliver APBI have evolved, using increasingly simple techniques that have encouraged dissemination of APBI to both large academic and small community practices. APBI may be administered using a variety of approaches, both invasive and noninvasive, and with the publication of single institutional protocols and a few small registry trials, APBI has begun to be used off protocol [3–6]. However, widespread adoption of external beam APBI, the most common technique in the United States, awaits the results of two recent randomized studies comparing whole breast irradiation to APBI, RAPID, and NSABP B-39 [7, 8].

5.2   Patient Selection

In 2009, with recognition of the increasing utilization of APBI, both the American Society for Therapeutic Radiation Oncology (ASTRO) and the Groupe Europeen de Curietherapie – European Society for Therapeutic Radiology and Oncology (GEC-ESTRO) published consensus guidelines to delineate clinically suitable/low-risk, cautionary/intermediate-risk, and unsuitable/high-risk categories for the receipt of APBI outside of a protocol [9, 10]. These guidelines were developed in the absence of randomized prospective data and to date, when evaluated clinically, have failed to show a relationship between consensus category and risk of local failure [11–13]. Consequently, variability exists regarding the utilization of APBI for specific patient groups, and subsequent guidelines from the American Society for Breast Surgeons (ASBrS) and the American Brachytherapy Society (ABS) differ from those published earlier (see Table 5.1 for comparison of "acceptable" patients by society) [14, 15]. Updated ASTRO consensus guidelines are expected in late 2016, but until their release, selecting a patient suitable for APBI outside of a study should be approached conservatively with APBI considered appropriate for postmenopausal patients with completely resected, pathologically staged T1 or small T2 tumors without regional lymph node involvement or multiple high-risk features including lymphovascular invasion or hormone receptor-negative status.

5.3   APBI Modality Selection

There are four main techniques for delivering APBI: (1) interstitial brachytherapy, (2) intracavity brachytherapy, (3) intraoperative radiation therapy (IORT), and (4) external beam radiation therapy (EBRT). The majority of APBI in the United States is currently delivered with EBRT, but the earliest techniques for APBI and the

Table 5.1 Consensus guidelines for APBI

	ASTRO (2009) "acceptable"	GEC-ESTRO (2009) "low risk"	ASBrS (2011)	ABS (2013)
Age (years)	≥60	>50	≥45 invasive ≥50 DCIS	≥50 years
Histology				
Size	≤2 cm	≤3 cm	≤3 cm	≤3 cm
Grade	Any	Any	a	a
Invasive lobular	No	No	Yes	Yes
DCIS	No	No	Yes	Yes
Multifocality	No	No	a	a
Multicentricity	No	No	a	a
EIC	No	No	a	a
LVI	No	No	a	No
ER/PR status	Positive	Any	a	Any
Surgical margins	≥2 mm	≥2 mm	"Negative"	"Negative"
Nodal status	pN0/pN0(i+)	pN0	pN0	"Negative"
Neoadjuvant therapy	Not allowed	Not allowed	a	a

[a]Indicates the lack of data or formal recommendation

technique with the most mature data is interstitial brachytherapy. Each of the four approaches was developed at different points in the evolution of APBI in an effort to improve on ease and conformality of treatment. As a result, their utilization differs widely based on physician expertise and institutional support. None of these techniques have been compared directly to detect differences in tumor control or toxicity, but each has their respective advantages and disadvantages.

In general, interstitial, intracavity, and IORT are more invasive techniques that require specialized equipment and additional physician and medical physics input compared to external beam radiation, but they can also be more convenient for patients by (1) expediting treatment delivery, (2) potentially decreasing skin toxicity, and (3) in the case of intraoperative radiation, obviating the need for multiple treatments. In contrast, external beam APBI is noninvasive and can be performed at nearly all radiation therapy centers without regard for additional equipment and technical training. Additionally, in contrast to IORT, it can also be pursued after final pathology is known and suitability for RT is fully evaluated thereby permitting for forward planning and superior dose homogeneity within the target volume.

5.4 Interstitial Brachytherapy

The delivery of interstitial brachytherapy represents the earliest practice of APBI and involves the surgical placement of approximately 10–20 interstitial catheters into the breast tissue following breast-conserving surgery. The procedure generally takes place once final pathology has returned to ensure that the patient is an appropriate candidate for APBI. At the time of interstitial placement, local anesthesia is

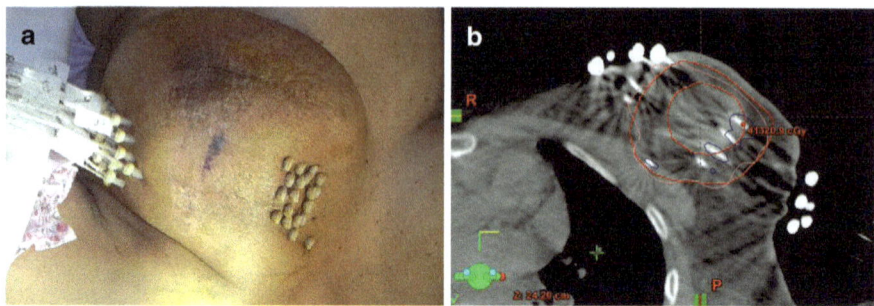

Fig. 5.1 Interstitial brachytherapy. (**a**) Demonstrates a photograph of a breast interstitial brachytherapy implant. (**b**) Depicts the axial non-contrast CT images of this patient's treatment plan (Courtesy of Atif Khan, MD)

administered, and the catheters, made of thin plastic tubing, are placed every 1–2 cm throughout the involved breast tissue to cover the tumor cavity with a 1–3 cm margin (Fig. 5.1). As with other interstitial brachytherapy procedures, a guide needle is placed within the catheter and inserted through the tissue at premarked locations at uniform depth and position. Once the guide needle has successfully penetrated the tissue and the catheter is in place, it is removed from the center of the catheter and repeated at each premarked position until all catheters are in position. Caps are then placed at the entry and exit points of each catheter for stabilization while also ensuring that the catheter extends adequately beyond the breast tissue to permit for connection to the brachytherapy delivery system. The patient then undergoes CT simulation; the lumpectomy cavity is delineated with a 1–2 cm margin, and planning is optimized to ensure conformal target coverage and dose homogeneity. Dose is delivered via low-dose rate (LDR) or high-dose rate (HDR) approaches, with a common dose fractionation scheme consisting of 45 Gy in 4.5 days (LDR) or 34 Gy in ten fractions (HDR). HDR dose constraints per NSABP B-39 include a ≥90% of target volume receiving ≥90% prescription dose while ensuring a breast tissue V150≤70 cc, V200≤20 cc, and a volume ratio of 1-(V150/V100) of ≥0.75. Additionally, <60% of the whole breast reference volume (excision cavity included) should receive ≥50% of prescription dose [16].

Long-term results from radiation therapy oncology group (RTOG) 95–17 and other studies have demonstrated a 10-year rate of ipsilateral breast tumor recurrence (IBTR) with interstitial brachytherapy of approximately 6% with good cosmetic results [17, 18]. However, this approach has waned in popularity due to the technical expertise and resources necessary to execute the treatment and has been largely replaced with less technically demanding methods.

5.5 Intracavitary Brachytherapy

As a procedurally simpler alternative to interstitial brachytherapy, intracavitary brachytherapy uses a single implantable device to deliver APBI. With intracavitary brachytherapy, a saline-filled balloon containing a single centrally placed catheter (e.g., MammoSite™, Contura™) or an ellipsis-shaped multicatheter device (e.g., Savvi™) is placed into the lumpectomy cavity following surgery (Fig. 5.2). The device may be placed immediately after lumpectomy at the time of surgery but is often placed days later when final pathology is known, in order to avoid a protracted period with the device in place or the need to remove the catheter if additional excisions are required. The catheter may be placed by either a breast surgeon or radiation oncologist and is introduced into the lumpectomy cavity through a percutaneous puncture site separate from the closed lumpectomy incision. The device is positioned to ensure a flush interface with all of the lumpectomy cavity walls as well as to achieve at least 5–7 mm distance from the skin surface. Following successful placement of the device, patients then undergo CT-based planning with contouring of the device surface in addition to delineation of the ipsilateral breast tissue and any trapped air or fluid outside the device. A clinical target volume (CTV) is then generated by a uniform 1 cm expansion around the device surface, limiting the expansion to 5 mm from the skin surface anteriorly and no further than the chest wall/pectoralis muscles posteriorly. No additional planning target volume (PTV) margin is added as the device will move with the target, so CTV is equivalent to PTV. Intracavitary brachytherapy can be administered using different dose and fractionation schemes, though a commonly utilized regimen is 34 Gy in ten fractions twice daily (BID) (Fig. 5.3). Treatment planning goals include at least 90 % of prescription dose covering ≥90 % of the target. The previously contoured air or fluid around the device is accounted for in this calculation, as it displaces a portion of the intended PTV. If the percentage of the PTV displaced by air or fluid exceeds 10 %, acceptable dose coverage is deemed not achievable. Additionally, per NSABP B-39 guidelines, the volume of tissue receiving 150 % of the dose should be ≤50 cc, and the volume of tissue receiving 200 % of the dose should be ≤10 cc. Less than 60 % of the whole breast reference volume minus the device volume should receive ≥50 % of prescription dose [16].

Once planning is complete, x-ray or ultrasound imaging prior to each treatment should be performed to ensure consistent device orientation. If unsatisfactory, repeat CT scan and planning should be pursued. Otherwise, if positioning is appropriate, an HDR source can be placed through the catheter(s) to deliver radiation, modifying position and dwell time as planned to ensure adequate dose to the entire cavity. This treatment approach results in a smaller amount of normal tissue exposure than other APBI techniques but may not offer the same conformality of dose seen with external beam treatments. Published data estimate 5-year ipsilateral breast tumor

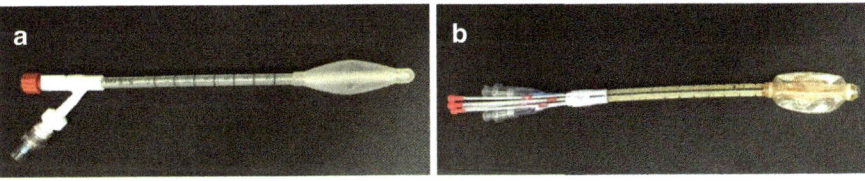

Fig. 5.2 Intracavitary brachytherapy devices. (**a**) Single lumen device. (**b**) Multilumen device (Courtesy of Jennifer Bellon, MD)

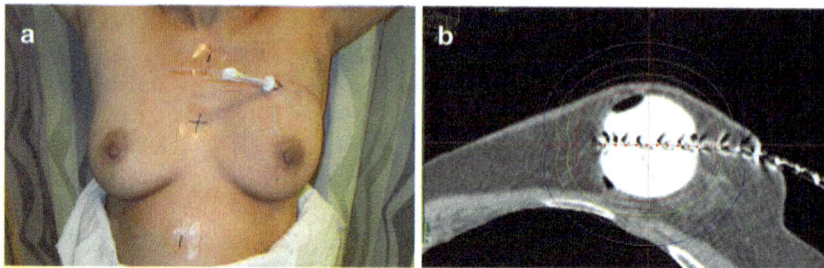

Fig. 5.3 Intracavitary brachytherapy treatment. (**a**) Demonstrates a photograph of a single lumen intracavitary brachytherapy device in place following lumpectomy. (**b**) Depicts the axial contrast CT images of a treatment plan (Courtesy of Atif Khan, MD and Phillip Devlin, MD)

recurrence (IBRT) rates of approximately 3–4 % [6]. Wound infection, seroma development, and/or explantation of the device due to malpositioning are also potential complications of this approach, although published rates in modern series differ [19, 20].

5.6   Intraoperative Radiation Therapy

Intraoperative radiation uses a linear accelerator (LINAC)-based treatment delivery system in the operating room following surgery to administer adjuvant radiation therapy in a single procedure. Following lumpectomy and prior to surgical closure of the lumpectomy cavity, either an electron applicator tube or a spherical kV applicator is placed directly into the lumpectomy cavity (Fig. 5.4). The LINAC then delivers a single high-dose fraction of radiation to the cavity and limited surrounding tissue. There is no formal target delineation and no dose optimization.

The use of intraoperative radiation (IORT) has been highlighted recently with the publication of the randomized TARGIT-A and ELIOT trials [21, 22]. In both trials, IORT was compared to adjuvant whole breast radiation. Together, these studies demonstrated the feasibility of IORT for APBI while also highlighting some of the challenges of an IORT approach. In the TARGIT-A trial, a 50 kV x-ray source was placed centrally within a spherical applicator. The applicator was then placed into the tumor bed, and 20 Gy of radiation was prescribed to the tumor bed surface over 20–35 min, with a dose of approximately 5–7 Gy delivered at 1 cm from the applicator. A single dose of 5 Gy is likely insufficient for tumor control, calling into question the adequacy of dose delivery. Additionally, external beam radiation therapy was administered after IORT if final pathology demonstrated higher risk disease than was anticipated, a situation experienced by more than 20 % of patients without final pathology at the time of IORT. At 5 years, IBRT in the IORT arm was significantly higher than in the WBRT arm (3.3 % vs. 1.3 %, p=0.042) but did meet prespecified criteria for noninferiority (absolute difference in recurrence of <2.5 %). As greater than 90 % of participants had estrogen receptor-positive cancers, characterized by low rates of local failure and a tendency for

Fig. 5.4 Intraoperative radiation. Figure demonstrates the setup for photon intraoperative radiation therapy (Courtesy of K Horst, MD)

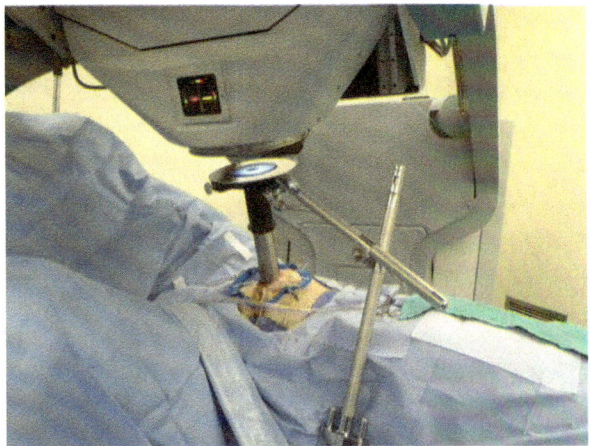

late recurrences; longer term follow-up is necessary to fully evaluate the noninferiority of APBI in this setting.

In the ELIOT trial, patients randomized to receive intraoperative radiation received 21 Gy in a single dose to the tumor bed, prescribed to the 90 % isodose using 6–9 MeV electrons via an applicator tube. Dose constraints ensured that ≤5 % of the heart and ≤20 % of the lung received <50 % of the dose, and no point in the contralateral breast received more than 15 % of the prescribed dose. The chest wall was selectively protected via lead or aluminum disks. For patients with high-risk features, as in the TARGIT-A trial, adjuvant whole breast radiation was administered following IORT. At 5 years, IBTR rate in the intraoperative arm was 4.4 % versus 0.4 % in the whole breast radiation group, meeting prespecified criteria for noninferiority (absolute recurrence rate for APBI <7.5 %). Fat necrosis rates were elevated with IORT, while acute skin toxicity and pulmonary fibrosis favored the IORT approach. Yet, when analyzed by clinicopathologic features, women with tumors exceeding 2 cm, those with more than four positive axillary lymph nodes, and those with high-grade disease or triple-negative subtype had risks of recurrence in excess of 10 %. This highlights the limitations of an up-front treatment approach and lends support for careful patient selection using current consensus guidelines for APBI.

5.7 External Beam Radiation Therapy

5.7.1 Patient Selection

In addition to those clinicopathologic factors included in the ASTRO consensus guidelines, physicians should also consider additional elements before selecting a patient for external beam APBI. First, the relative size of the lumpectomy site compared to the size of the involved breast at the time of postoperative physical

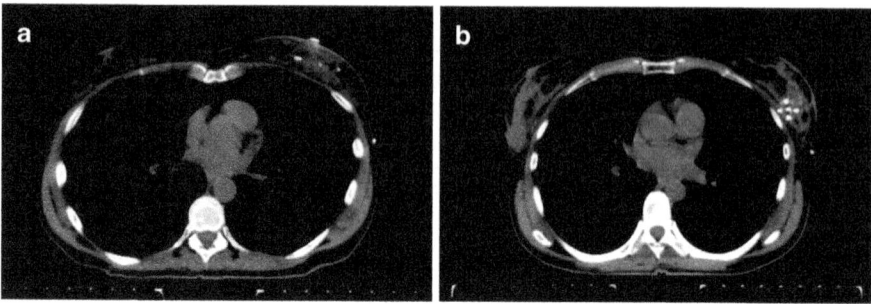

Fig. 5.5 Comparison of lumpectomy cavity. (**a**) Depicts axial noncontrast CT images of a patient with surgical clips placed in the lumpectomy cavity to assist with target delineation. (**b**) Depicts axial noncontrast CT images of a different patient with a radiopaque device positioned in the lumpectomy cavity for target delineation

examination should be favorable, such that a majority of the breast would not be encompassed in the eventual planning target volume (PTV). A lumpectomy PTV/breast ratio greater than 25–35 % can result in an undesired cosmetic outcome (for additional specific constraints, see Sect. 5.7.4) [23]. In addition to the lumpectomy to breast ratio, several other factors have been associated with a poor cosmetic outcome following external beam APBI compared to whole breast irradiation. These include older patient age, active smoking status, tumors located in the central or inner quadrant, and large seromas [24].

Prior to committing a patient to external beam APBI treatment, the treating physician should ensure that the collaborating breast surgeon has placed clips intraoperatively to delineate the lumpectomy cavity. Using the seroma alone to determine the location of the tumor is unreliable as the size and configuration of the seroma change with time. Studies have suggested that inter-physician agreement in defining the surgical bed improves with an increasing number of clips and that six or more clips significantly increase the accuracy of tumor bed delineation [25, 26]. Alternatively, there are bioabsorbable, radiopaque devices that can be sutured to the walls of the resection cavity at the time of lumpectomy to assist in delineating the tumor bed (Fig. 5.5) [27].

5.7.2 Simulation

On the day of simulation, the patient is placed supine or prone (depending on approach, see Sect. 5.7.4 for details) on a breast board. If supine, a radiopaque wire is placed around the extent of the palpable breast tissue to delineate the whole breast volume. A second wire is placed over the incision to identify the surgical scar. Axial noncontrast CT images are obtained in 2.5 mm thick slices, superiorly from the angle of the mandible through the lung bases, except for the region of the resection cavity, where slice thickness is narrowed to 1.25 mm to ensure precision in identifying the seroma. Following the initial scan, a review of the CT images is performed to ensure that clips are present in the vicinity of the surgical cavity. Tattoos are then placed in the same number and configuration as those for traditional whole breast treatments.

5.7.3   Target Delineation

Following simulation, target volumes and organs at risks (OARs) are then identified and contoured. The target volumes include the breast, lumpectomy cavity, lumpectomy CTV, and lumpectomy PTV (Table 5.2, Fig. 5.6). The OARs include the heart and bilateral lungs. For assistance with contours, the RTOG breast atlas can be accessed at www.rtog.org/CoreLab/ContouringAtlases/BreastCancerAtlas.aspx [28]. For APBI cases, accuracy in identifying the lumpectomy cavity is vital, and all available information, including preoperative imaging and the operative report, should be utilized.

5.7.4   Treatment Planning

APBI can be administered with patients in either the supine or prone positions. There are two common supine APBI planning techniques, a three-field technique and a technique using multiple non coplanar beams. The three-field technique consists of

Table 5.2 Contouring definitions for external beam treatment planning

Target volumes	Description
Breast	The breast contour should include all glandular tissue evident on CT with wiring at the time of simulation assisting with the definition of clinical anatomic borders Cranial: below the head of the clavicle at the insertion of the second rib Caudal: the loss of breast tissue Medial: ipsilateral sternal edge Lateral: midaxillary line permitting for breast ptosis Anterior: skin or a few millimeters deep to the skin (for dose evaluation) Posterior: anterior to the pectoralis muscles and chest wall
Lumpectomy cavity	The lumpectomy cavity is contoured on axial CT images and confirmed using the coronal and sagittal planes. It should include any visible seroma and associated soft tissue changes from surgery and all clips placed in the resection cavity at the time of the operation. For lumpectomy cavities deep in the breast or those located close to the chest wall, the entire operative track from the cavity to the skin should not be included. When the extent of the resection cavity is in doubt, comparison with the soft tissue of the contralateral breast can be helpful. This volume should not extend beyond the breast tissue
Lumpectomy CTV	Lumpectomy cavity + 1.0–1.5 cm expansion, respecting anatomic boundaries
Lumpectomy PTV	Lumpectomy CTV + 0.5–1.0 cm expansion, may extend outside the patient surface and/or into the chest wall or ipsilateral lung

Fig. 5.6 APBI contours. Figure shows the target volumes and organs at risk for APBI including the lumpectomy cavity (*red*), CTV with 1.5 cm expansion (*pink*), CTV with 2.0 cm expansion (*purple*), breast (*green*), left lung (*orange*), and right lung (*yellow*)

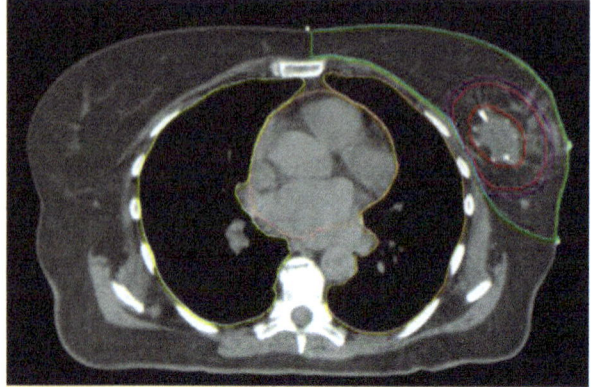

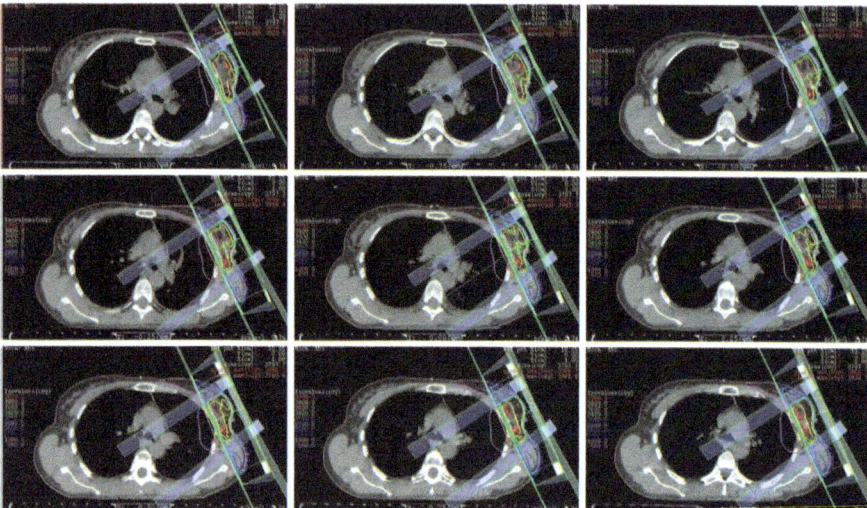

Fig. 5.7 Three-field technique. Figure depicts an APBI plan using mini-tangents and an en face electron field. The *green line* represents the 95 % isodose line (IDL)

two mini-tangents and a single enface electron field (Fig. 5.7). The isocenter is placed in the approximate center of the resection cavity at the time of CT simulation to avoid undue shifts. Then, the parallel-opposed photon field angles are selected to limit exposure to the OARs and uninvolved breast tissue. The electron setup point is then positioned to intersect with the photon isocenter, and the field is positioned en face. A margin of 0.7 cm to block edge accounts for penumbra. Multileaf collimators shape the photon field apertures, and Cerrobend blocking defines the electron field. With this approach, the tangent fields are generally weighted equally and collectively account for approximately 80 % of the dose, with the remaining 20 % of the dose delivered en face. However, differential weighting as well as noncoplanar photon fields may be used as needed to achieve prescription goals.

Table 5.3 Treatment constraints for external beam treatment planning

Organs at risk	Constraints
Ipsilateral lung	V20<3% V10<10% V5<20%
Contralateral lung	V20<1% V10<2% V5<3%
Contralateral breast	<3% of prescription dose to any point
Heart	As low as reasonably achievable, making efforts to avoid cardiac structures entirely
Thyroid	Maximum point dose ≤3% of prescription dose

At Massachusetts General Hospital (MGH), dose has traditionally been 36 Gy in nine fractions of 4 Gy delivered twice daily (BID) or 40 Gy in ten fractions of 4 Gy delivered once daily. However, a more widely employed dose/fractionation scheme, as adopted in both the NSABP B-39 and RAPID trials, utilizes 38.5 Gy in ten fractions of 3.85 Gy BID over 5–10 days [7, 8].

Using the dose fractionation schemes above, the goal is to cover 98% of the PTV with 95% of the prescription dose while limiting the ratio of PTV to total ipsilateral breast tissue to less than 25%, the nontarget breast tissue volume minus PTV receiving 50% of the prescription dose to less than 50%, and the total ipsilateral breast tissue receiving 50% of the prescription dose to less than 60%. Constraints on OARs are also more conservative than those used for whole breast treatments (Table 5.3) [16, 29]. In rare circumstances when the heart dose remains unacceptably high, deep inspiration breathhold may be considered to achieve the desired metrics.

The second method of delivering APBI in the supine position consists of multiple, often four, noncoplanar fields, made up of a combination of left and right superior-to-inferior and inferior-to-superior obliques (Fig. 5.8). Beam weighting is optimized to ensure that the PTV is encompassed by the 95% isodose line (IDL) while ensuring a hotspot <110%. The ipsilateral breast volume is limited to ensure that no more than 25–35% receives 100% of the prescription dose. Prescription dose and OAR constraints are in keeping with those detailed above [30].

In contrast, patients treated in the prone position generally receive treatment using a mini-tangent field arrangement, though noncoplanar approaches can also be employed (Fig. 5.9). Traditionally, the dose used with this technique consists of 30 Gy over five fractions of 6 Gy administered every other day, and in this setting, 100% of the PTV should receive 95% of the dose with no greater than 60% of the breast volume receiving 50% of prescription dose [31]. However, patient positioning is the unique factor in this case, and both the prescription dose and dosimetric constraints could reasonably be interchanged with the supine techniques detailed above.

Finally, there is limited research on the delivery of APBI with proton beam radiation. Early work using 3D conformal proton beam radiation with 1–3 fields resulted

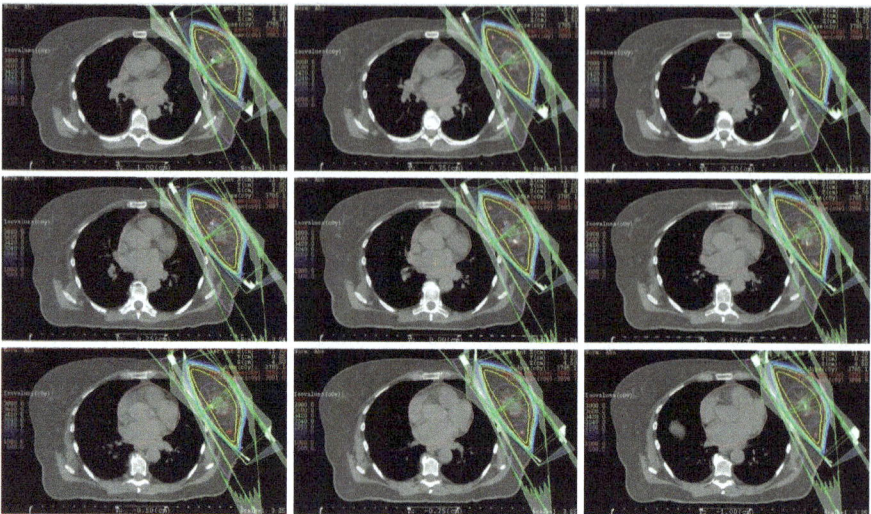

Fig. 5.8 Multiple noncoplanar beam technique. Figure depicts an APBI plan using four noncoplanar photon beams. The *green line* represents the 95 % isodose line (IDL)

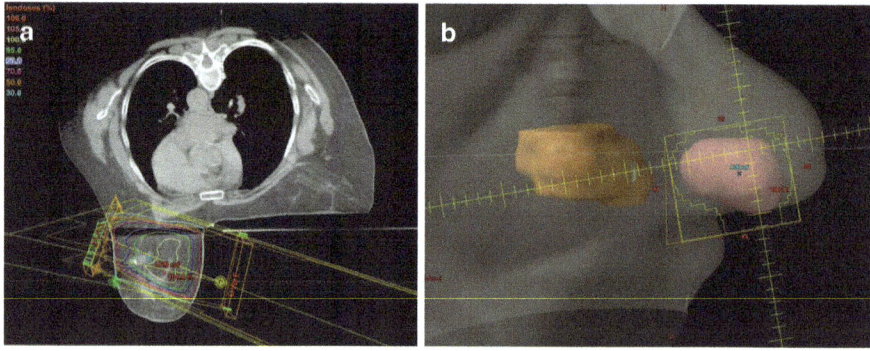

Fig. 5.9 Prone technique. (**a**) Depicts an APBI plan using mini-tangents with the patient in the prone position. (**b**) Shows the beams eye view of this technique with sparing of the heart and superior breast tissue (Courtesy of Raymond Mailhot, MD)

in unacceptable cosmesis including telangiectasias and pigmentation changes, but other studies using multiple fields with skin-sparing approaches or proton beam scanning have suggested more favorable cosmetic outcomes [32, 33]. Proton beam radiation can be delivered with the patient either supine or prone, and additional research is warranted. However, given both the cost of proton beam radiation and the limited access to proton beam facilities, consideration of the cost to benefit ratio for each patient is necessary.

Determining the ideal treatment technique for each patient is based on multiple factors including the patient's anatomy, the size and location of the lumpectomy cavity within the breast, and the treating team's experience using each of the above methods. In general, the three-field technique is the simplest to plan for those new to APBI because of its similarity to whole breast treatment techniques but may not be appropriate for patients with lumpectomy cavities that are lateralized to the extremes of the breast tissue, either far medially in proximity to the heart and contralateral breast or far laterally approximating the axilla where total breast dose constraints may be difficult to achieve and an en face field would not be technically deliverable, due to cone table interference. In these circumstances, a noncoplanar beam technique may be superior. However, a noncoplanar beam technique may be less useful for patients with lumpectomy cavities in the far superior breast where noncoplanar fields could generate high lung metrics or among patients with a short neck when beam entry or exit could result in dose to the chin/face. Finally, the prone technique is of value among patients with pendulous breasts where a supine approach would result in the potential for more uninvolved breast tissue exposure and/or when the seroma is in proximity to the heart or lungs. It would be less useful in patients with far lateral seromas close to the chest wall or among those with truncal obesity or orthopedic conditions for whom reproducibility and tolerability of setup would be in question.

5.7.5 Position Verification

Once planning is complete, the targeted approach of APBI necessitates accurate and precise positioning of the patient. As the breast is a superficial, soft tissue structure, its position may vary in relation to bony anatomy with each setup, and therefore, accurate tracking with organ-focused imaging is imperative. In a study evaluating different alignment approaches, both laser alignment and bony anatomy alignment have been found to be insufficient for ensuring the level of accuracy needed, with errors in setup exceeding 5 mm using either approach [34, 35]. In contrast, the use of surface imaging and clip alignment has been found to minimize target registration errors. Much of the work on surface imaging has utilized AlignRT™, an imaging system consisting of two three-dimensional (3D) high-resolution cameras that are mounted on the ceiling of the treatment room and acquire images of the patient in treatment position prior to each fraction. AlignRT™ uses image gating to capture the 3D data at a consistent point in the patient's breathing cycle. Once obtained, it is then referenced to the patient's planning CT anatomy using surface-matching software. Comparisons of the images are generated, and any necessary couch shifts are displayed for the radiation therapists along with new couch coordinates to confer optimal positioning (Fig. 5.10). Studies of this technique have estimated setup errors of approximately 3 mm when used alone. With the addition of orthogonal films aligned to internal surgical clips prior to each fraction target, registration errors can be minimized to within 1 mm of desired setup. Therefore one or both of these techniques should be utilized as available to ensure accuracy and consistency with each fraction [35] (Fig. 5.11).

Fig. 5.10 External beam
patient setup verification
with AlignRT™. Figure
depicts an AlignRT™
image overlaying the
patient reference image
(*purple*) to the daily
monitoring surface (*green*)
along with the required
shifts necessary for
alignment of the two
images (Courtesy of David
Gierga, PhD)

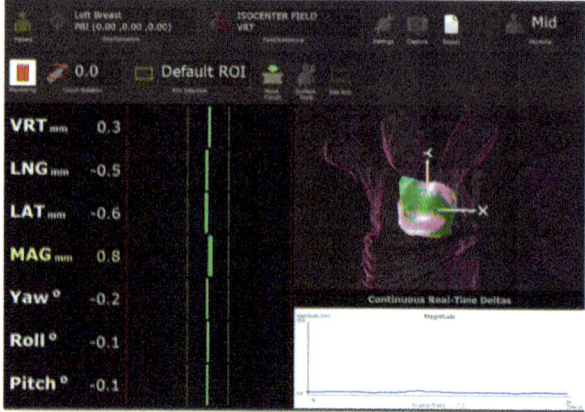

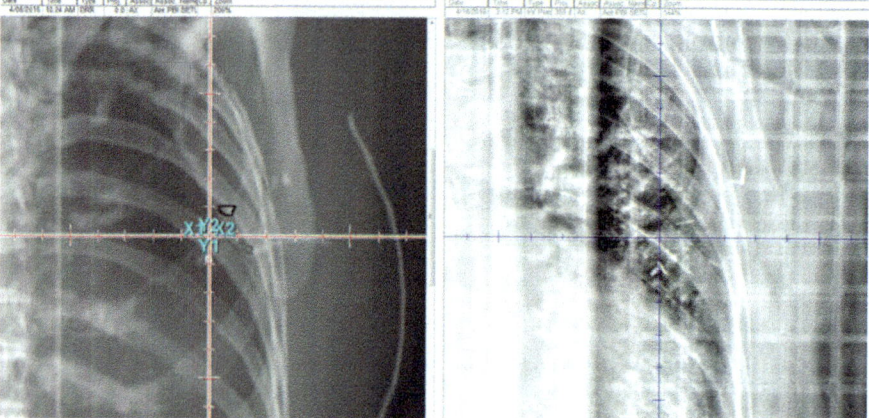

Fig. 5.11 External beam patient setup verification with clip matching. Figure shows a comparison of a patient digitally reconstructed radiograph (DRR) with clips outlined in black with the patient's daily setup image. The two are compared, and shifts are performed to ensure clip positioning of the daily setup matches that of the DRR (Courtesy of David Gierga, PhD)

Conclusion

Accelerated partial breast irradiation is a valuable treatment technique that obviates the need for long treatment courses and unnecessary radiation exposure. Care should be taken, not only in selecting the proper patient for this technique but in ensuring accuracy at each stage of planning. Until mature randomized data or updated consensus guidelines are available, candidates for APBI off protocol should be limited to those who fit the suitability criteria as detailed by either the current ASTRO/GEC-ESTRO or ASBrS/ABS consensus statements. Consensus guidelines suggest which patients are eligible for APBI, but they are not a replacement for clinical judgment, and physicians should take care to consider the wisdom of using APBI on a patient-by-patient basis. From this perspective, it is necessary to evaluate the patient's anatomy and comorbidities as both can impact treatment feasibility, complications, and long-term cosmesis. To date, none of the four APBI techniques discussed above have been compared in a randomized fashion, and most individual studies of APBI report comparable rates of local failure, so if APBI is considered appropriate, technique will be determined as much by the clinicopathologic factors above as by the modality with which the treating physician has the most facility. In the current era, interstitial brachytherapy is rarely used, having been supplanted by intracavitary and external beam radiation therapy. Both require less technical expertise on the part of the treating physician and afford precise forward planning with the use of 3D imaging. Newer techniques using proton beam scanning radiation are also under investigation. In all, APBI has potential to become the standard of care for early-stage, low-risk breast cancer patients, and the field awaits the publication of the RAPID and NSABP B-39 trials to provide the much needed data.

References

1. Fisher B, Anderson S, Bryant J et al (2002) Twenty-year follow-up of a randomized trial comparing total mastectomy, lumpectomy, and lumpectomy plus irradiation for the treatment of invasive breast cancer. N Engl J Med 347(16):1233–1241
2. Early Breast Cancer Trialists' Collaborative Group (1995) Effects of radiotherapy and surgery in early breast cancer. An overview of the randomized trials. N Engl J Med 333(22):1444–1455
3. Vicini F, Winter K, Wong J, Pass H, Rabinovitch R, Chafe S et al (2010) Initial efficacy results of RTOG 0319: three-dimensional conformal radiation therapy (3D-CRT) confined to the region of the lumpectomy cavity for stage I/II breast carcinoma. Int J Radiat Oncol Biol Phys 77(4):1120–1127
4. Formenti SC, Hsu H, Fenton-Kerimian M, Roses D, Guth A, Jozsef G et al (2012) Prone accelerated partial breast irradiation after breast-conserving surgery: five-year results of 100 patients. Int J Radiat Oncol Biol Phys 84(3):606–611
5. Shah C, Wilkinson JB, Lanni T, Jawad M, Wobb J, Fowler A et al (2013) Five-year outcomes and toxicities using 3-dimensional conformal external beam radiation therapy to deliver accelerated partial breast irradiation. Clin Breast Cancer 13(3):206–211
6. Shah C, Badiyan S, Ben Wilkinson J, Vicini F, Beitsch P, Keisch M et al (2013) Treatment efficacy with accelerated partial breast irradiation (APBI): final analysis of the American Society of Breast Surgeons MammoSite® breast brachytherapy registry trial. Ann Surg Oncol 20(10):3279–3285
7. Olivotto IA, Whelan TJ, Parpia S, Kim DH, Berrang T, Truong PT et al (2013) Interim cosmetic and toxicity results from RAPID: a randomized trial of accelerated partial breast irradiation using three-dimensional conformal external beam radiation therapy. J Clin Oncol 31(32):4038–4045
8. NSABP (2006) B-39, RTOG 0413: a Randomized Phase III Study of conventional whole breast irradiation versus partial breast irradiation for women with stage 0, I, or II breast cancer. Clin Adv Hematol Oncol 4(10):719–721
9. Smith BD, Arthur DW, Buchholz TA, Haffty BG, Hahn CA, Hardenbergh PH et al (2009) Accelerated partial breast irradiation consensus statement from the American Society for Radiation Oncology (ASTRO). Int J Radiat Oncol Biol Phys 74(4):987–1001
10. Polgár C, Van Limbergen E, Pötter R, Kovács G, Polo A, Lyczek J et al (2010) GEC-ESTRO breast cancer working group. Patient selection for accelerated partial-breast irradiation (APBI)

after breast-conserving surgery: recommendations of the Groupe Européen de Curiethérapie-European Society for Therapeutic Radiology and Oncology (GEC-ESTRO) breast cancer working group based on clinical evidence (2009). Radiother Oncol 94(3):264–273

11. Beitsch P, Vicini F, Keisch M, Haffty B, Shaitelman S, Lyden M (2010) Five-year outcome of patients classified in the "unsuitable" category using the American Society of Therapeutic Radiology and Oncology (ASTRO) Consensus Panel guidelines for the application of accelerated partial breast irradiation: an analysis of patients treated on the American Society of Breast Surgeons MammoSite® Registry trial. Ann Surg Oncol 17(Suppl 3):219–225

12. Wilkinson JB, Beitsch PD, Shah C, Arthur D, Haffty BG, Wazer DE et al (2013) Evaluation of current consensus statement recommendations for accelerated partial breast irradiation: a pooled analysis of William Beaumont Hospital and American Society of Breast Surgeon MammoSite Registry Trial Data. Int J Radiat Oncol Biol Phys 85(5):1179–1185

13. Stull TS, Catherine Goodwin M, Gracely EJ, Chernick MR, Carella RJ, Frazier TG et al (2012) A single-institution review of accelerated partial breast irradiation in patients considered "cautionary" by the American Society for Radiation Oncology. Ann Surg Oncol 19(2):553–559

14. Consensus statement for accelerated partial breast irradiation from the American Society of Breast Surgeons: https://www.breastsurgeons.org/new_layout/about/statements/PDF_Statements/APBI.pdf

15. Shah C, Vicini F, Wazer DE, Arthur D, Patel RR (2013) The American Brachytherapy Society consensus statement for accelerated partial breast irradiation. Brachytherapy 12:267–277

16. NSABP B-39/RTOG 0413 protocol: http://atc.wustl.edu/protocols/nsabp/b-39/0413.pdf

17. Rabinovitch R, Winter K, Kuske R, Bolton J, Arthur D, Scroggins T et al (2014) RTOG 95–17, a Phase II trial to evaluate brachytherapy as the sole method of radiation therapy for Stage I and II breast carcinoma--year-5 toxicity and cosmesis. Brachytherapy 13(1):17–22

18. Polgár C, Fodor J, Major T, Sulyok Z, Kásler M (2013) Breast-conserving therapy with partial or whole breast irradiation: ten-year results of the Budapest randomized trial. Radiother Oncol 108(2):197–202

19. Niehoff P, Polgár C, Ostertag H, Major T, Sulyok Z, Kimmig B et al (2006) Clinical experience with the MammoSite radiation therapy system for brachytherapy of breast cancer: results from an international phase II trial. Radiother Oncol 79(3):316–320

20. Shah C, Khwaja S, Badiyan S, Wilkinson JB, Vicini FA, Beitsch P et al (2013) Brachytherapy-based partial breast irradiation is associated with low rates of complications and excellent cosmesis. Brachytherapy 12(4):278–284

21. Vaidya JS, Wenz F, Bulsara M, Tobias JS, Joseph DJ, Keshtgar M et al (2014) Risk-adapted targeted intraoperative radiotherapy versus whole-breast radiotherapy for breast cancer: 5-year results for local control and overall survival from the TARGIT-A randomised trial. Lancet 383(9917):603–613

22. Veronesi U, Orecchia R, Maisonneuve P, Viale G, Rotmensz N, Sangalli C et al (2013) Intraoperative radiotherapy versus external radiotherapy for early breast cancer (ELIOT): a randomised controlled equivalence trial. Lancet Oncol 14(13):1269–1277

23. Leonard KL, Hepel JT, Hiatt JR, Dipetrillo TA, Price LL, Wazer DE (2013) The effect of dose-volume parameters and interfraction interval on cosmetic outcome and toxicity after 3-dimensional conformal accelerated partial breast irradiation. Int J Radiat Oncol Biol Phys 85(3):623–629

24. Peterson D, Truong PT, Parpia S, Olivotto IA, Berrang T, Kim DH et al (2015) Predictors of adverse cosmetic outcome in the RAPID trial: an exploratory analysis. Int J Radiat Oncol Biol Phys 91(5):968–976

25. Shaikh T, Chen T, Khan A, Yue NJ, Kearney T, Cohler A et al (2010) Improvement in interobserver accuracy in delineation of the lumpectomy cavity using fiducial markers. Int J Radiat Oncol Biol Phys 78(4):1127–1134

26. Ippolito E, Trodella L, Silipigni S, D'Angelillo RM, Di Donato A, Fiore M et al (2014) Estimating the value of surgical clips for target volume delineation in external beam partial breast radiotherapy. Clin Oncol (R Coll Radiol) 26(11):677–683

27. Cross MJ, Ross J, Jones S, Smith A, Beck T (2015) Implantable marker to facilitate use of hypofractionated radiation in early breast cancer. J Clin Oncol 33(Suppl 28S):abstr 38
28. RTOG breast contouring atlas: http://www.rtog.org/CoreLab/ContouringAtlases/BreastCancerAtlas.aspx
29. Recht A, Ancukiewicz M, Alm El-Din MA, Lu XQ, Martin C, Berman SM et al (2009) Lung dose-volume parameters and the risk of pneumonitis for patients treated with accelerated partial-breast irradiation using three-dimensional conformal radiotherapy. J Clin Oncol 27(24):3887–3893
30. Baglan KL, Sharpe MB, Jaffray D, Frazier RC, Fayad J, Kestin LL et al (2003) Accelerated partial breast irradiation using 3D conformal radiation therapy (3D-CRT). Int J Radiat Oncol Biol Phys 55(2):302–311
31. Formenti SC, Truong MT, Goldberg JD, Mukhi V, Rosenstein B, Roses D et al (2004) Prone accelerated partial breast irradiation after breast-conserving surgery: preliminary clinical results and dose-volume histogram analysis. Int J Radiat Oncol Biol Phys 60(2):493–504
32. Galland-Girodet S, Pashtan I, MacDonald SM, Ancukiewicz M, Hirsch AE, Kachnic LA et al (2014) Long-term cosmetic outcomes and toxicities of proton beam therapy compared with photon-based 3-dimensional conformal accelerated partial-breast irradiation: a phase 1 trial. Int J Radiat Oncol Biol Phys 90(3):493–500
33. Bush DA, Do S, Lum S, Garberoglio C, Mirshahidi H, Patyal B, Grove R et al (2014) Partial breast radiation therapy with proton beam: 5-year results with cosmetic outcomes. Int J Radiat Oncol Biol Phys 90(3):501–505
34. Bert C, Metheany KG, Doppke KP et al (2006) Clinical experience with a 3D surface patient setup system for alignment of partial-breast irradiation patients. Int J Radiat Oncol Biol Phys 64:1265–1274
35. Gierga DP, Riboldi M, Turcotte JC, Sharp GC, Jiang SB, Taghian AG et al (2008) Comparison of target registration errors for multiple image-guided techniques in accelerated partial breast irradiation. Int J Radiat Oncol Biol Phys 70(4):1239–1246

Deep Inspiration Breath Hold

6

Carmen Bergom, Adam Currey, An Tai,
and Jonathan B. Strauss

Contents

6.1 Rationale for Deep Inspiration Breath Hold

The use of radiotherapy in the postmastectomy setting or as part of breast-conserving therapy improves local control and overall survival [17, 18]. However, the breast cancer-specific survival advantage for patients receiving radiation therapy may be partially negated by higher non-breast cancer mortality [16, 31], which may be due to cardiac mortality [7, 11, 13, 14, 29]. Patients with left-sided breast cancer receiving radiation had increased cardiac mortality [29, 61], and the rates of major coronary events [14, 70] and cardiac deaths [25, 70] increased with extrapolated mean heart radiation dose. Patients receiving internal mammary chain (IMC) radiation [32] and patients treated with left-sided breast conservation therapy [26] also

C. Bergom, MD, PhD (✉) • A. Currey, MD • A. Tai, PhD
Department of Radiation Oncology, Medical College of Wisconsin, Milwaukee, WI, USA
e-mail: cbergom@mcw.edu

J.B. Strauss, MD
Department of Radiation Oncology, Northwestern University Feinberg School of Medicine, Chicago, IL, USA

© Springer International Publishing Switzerland 2016
J.R. Bellon et al. (eds.), *Radiation Therapy Techniques and Treatment Planning for Breast Cancer*, Practical Guides in Radiation Oncology,
DOI 10.1007/978-3-319-40392-2_6

demonstrated higher late cardiac morbidity. The increase in cardiac morbidity and mortality related to radiation therapy is influenced by the presence of other cardiac risk factors as well as the use of adjuvant chemotherapy [26, 32, 63]. However, the interactions of these other non-radiation factors are not always supra-additive [14].

The evidence for increased levels of cardiac morbidity and mortality includes many studies from patients treated prior to the mid-1980s [7, 13, 31, 61]. Over time, advances in radiotherapy such as three-dimensional conformal radiation therapy (3DCRT) have reduced the doses of radiation received by the heart; breast cancer radiation treatments in more modern eras have lower excess cardiac mortality [13, 15, 29, 31]. Techniques such as prone breast radiation [22] and proton therapy [2, 43] have been demonstrated to decrease cardiac radiation doses in some patients. Intensity-modulated radiation therapy (IMRT) may decrease the amount of heart tissue that receives high doses of radiation, but it may increase the amount of heart tissue receiving low radiation doses [42].

Deep inspiration breath hold (DIBH) is another tool radiation oncologists use to reduce dose to the heart. This technique exploits the increase in the separation of the heart and the chest wall when the lung expands with inspiration in order to decrease the radiation doses received by the heart. The patient takes and holds a breath within a specified threshold during radiation, effectively minimizing the heart radiation dose and volume using tangential radiation (Figs. 6.1 and 6.2) [40]. DIBH serves as an alternative to prone breast irradiation for left-sided breast cancers [74] and is also suitable for use with prone breast irradiation [47].

Treatment of the IMC lymph nodes results in an increase in heart dose versus treatment of the breast or chest wall alone [9]. IMC nodal treatment is controversial [28, 73], but the recent MA.20 [79] and EORTC 22922 [54] studies demonstrating benefits for the addition of regional nodal radiotherapy included treatment of the IMC nodes. Rates of IMC nodal radiotherapy may therefore increase. It has been estimated that there is a 4–7.4 % increase in heart disease and/or major coronary events for each 1 Gy in mean heart dose [14, 62], with no minimum threshold. Thus, minimizing the doses and volumes of irradiated heart with breast cancer radiotherapy is important to limit cardiac morbidity and mortality.

6.2   DIBH Techniques

Two main methods to obtain DIBH are voluntary DIBH (vDIBH) and moderate DIBH using spirometry-based active breathing coordinator or active breathing control (ABC) devices [81] (e.g., ABC from Elekta, Stockholm, Sweden). A technical challenge with DIBH is the inter- and intrafractional reproducibility of patient geometry and anatomy. ABC devices may reduce this variability. ABC yields reproducible immobilization of the chest wall by monitoring the breathing cycle and facilitating a breath hold at a defined lung volume by stopping the flow of air at a prespecified volume for a predefined period of time (Fig. 6.3) [57, 58, 81]. ABC reduced radiation doses to the heart (Table 6.1) and high intrafractional setup reproducibility has been reported, with one study demonstrating setup errors of

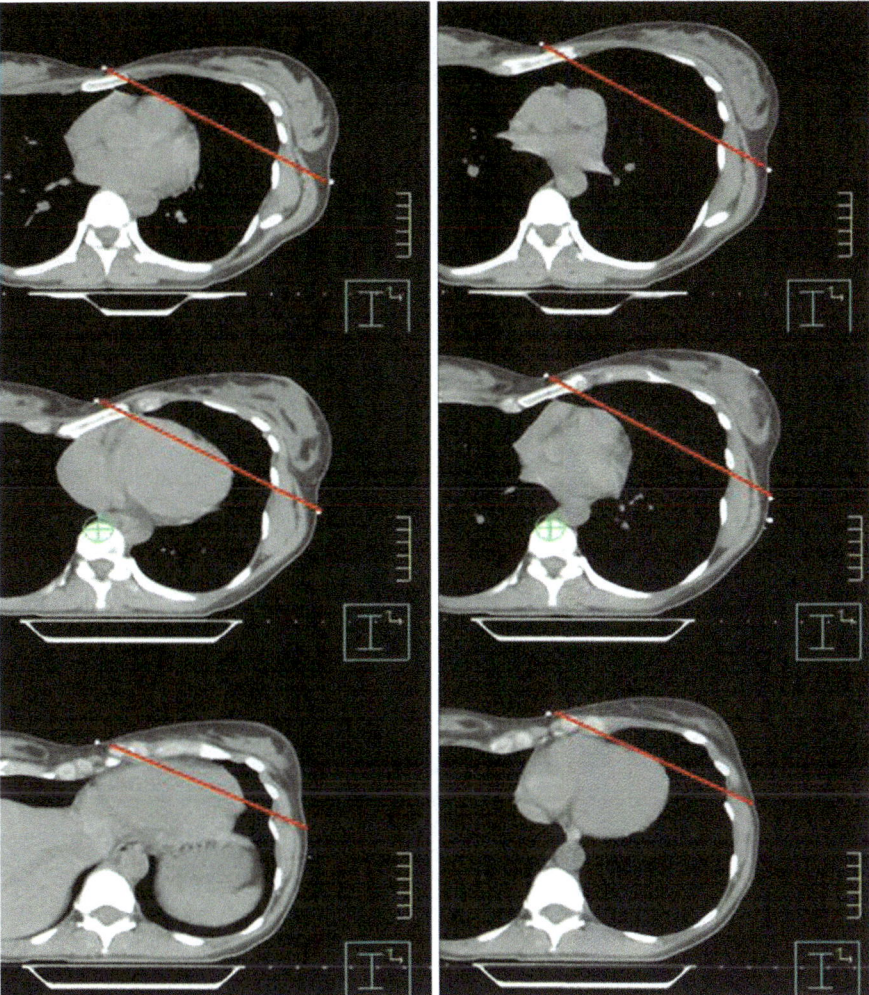

Fig. 6.1 Free breathing and DIBH axial CT images illustrate potential improvements in heart radiation exposure with tangential breast radiation treatment. The cardiac position in the same patient is shown at free breathing (*left*) and in DIBH (*right*) at three comparable axial vertebral body levels on CT. The *red line* represents a potential tangent field

approximately 1 mm and always less than 2 mm, as measured on electronic portal images [57].

In contrast to the ABC method, for vDIBH patients are instructed to perform deep inspiration and the respiratory motion is typically monitored using one of several methods. For example, in a common vDIBH technique, the vertical displacement of an external surrogate at the sternum or abdomen provides a relative inspiration level compared to the patient's baseline breathing with a real-time positioning management system (RPM) (e.g., from Varian Medical Systems, Inc., Palo

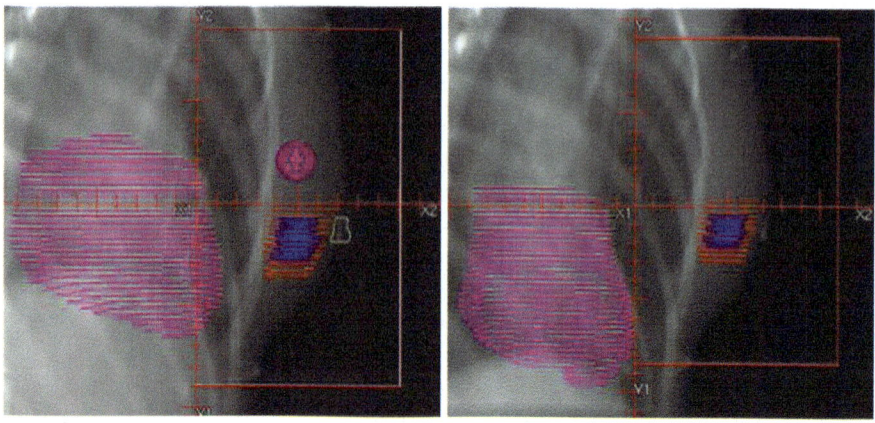

Fig. 6.2 Digitally reconstructed radiographs from a patient in free breathing and DIBH highlights the more favorable position of the heart for treatment. An expansion of the lumpectomy bed to CTV is outlined in *red*. The heart is contoured in *purple*. Note the distance from the lumpectomy bed to the heart between the free breathing (*left*) and deep inspiration (*right*)

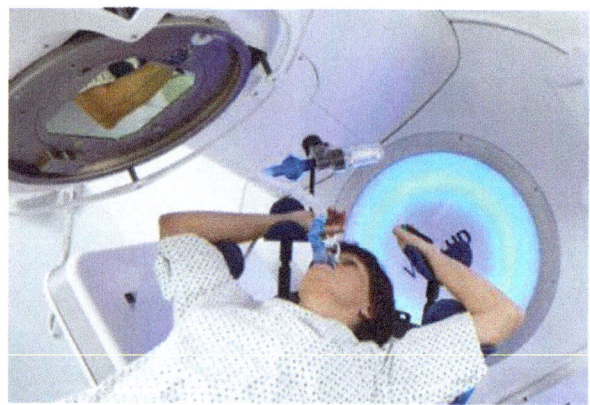

Fig. 6.3 An ABC breathing device for DIBH. A switch is held in the right hand which is pressed during the breath hold and can be released if the patient feels uncomfortable (Photo courtesy of Elekta)

Alto, CA, USA). This system generates sinusoidal tracings of the surrogate over time that serve as a proxy for chest excursion (Fig. 6.4). However, for this method and ABC DIBH, treatment is not gated or monitored based upon the targeted breast or chest wall position. In optical tracking systems (e.g., AlignRT, Vision RT Ltd, London, UK; Sentinel, C-RAD, Uppsala, Sweden) [39], stereovision is used to reconstruct the three-dimensional surface of the patient, visualizing the alignment of the reference surface and the reconstructed surface at the region of interest to provide real-time positioning (Fig. 6.5) [1, 52, 60]. Betgen et al. [4] performed vDIBH using an optical surface tracking system. After setup corrections, variations

Table 6.1 Published comparisons of dose reductions in heart and LAD doses using DIBH techniques

Study	DIBH method	# Patients	Area(s) treated	Mean heart dose (Gy)			Mean LAD dose (Gy)		
				FB	DIBH	Reduction with DIBH	FB	DIBH	Reduction with DIBH
Wang et al. [77]	ABC	20	Breast	3.2	1.3	59%	20.0	5.9	71%
Mast et al. [45]	ABC	20	Breast	3.3 2.7	1.8 1.5	45%[a] 44%[b]	18.6 14.9	9.6 6.7	48%[a] 55%[b]
Nissen and Appelt [49]	ABC	227[c]	Breast/CW ± SCV + Ax LN	5.2	2.7	48%	–	–	–
Swanson et al. [67]	ABC	87	Breast/CW ± SCV + Ax LN	4.2	2.5	40%	–	–	–
Comsa et al. [12]	ABC	20 30	Breast ± boost Breast/CW + SCV + Ax LN	3.1 4.5	1.2 2.1	61% 53%	– –	– –	– –
Eldredge-Hindy et al. [20]	ABC	86	Breast ± boost ± SCV + Ax ± IMC LN	2.7	0.9	67%[d]	–	–	–
Stranzl and Zurl [65]	vDIBH (RPM)	22	Breast/CW ± boost	2.3	1.3	44%	–	–	–
Stranzl et al. [66]	vDIBH (RPM)	11	Breast/CW + IMC LN	4.0	2.5	38%	–	–	–
Borst et al. [6]	vDIBH (other)	19	Breast/CW ± boost	5.1	1.7	67%	11.4	5.5	52%
Johansen et al. [36]	vDIBH (RPM)	16	Breast	6.5	2.5	62%	–	–	–
McIntosh et al. [46]	vDIBH (RPM)	10	Breast	Not reported	Not reported	48%	Not reported	Not reported	43%

(continued)

Table 6.1 (continued)

Study	DIBH method	# Patients	Area(s) treated	Mean heart dose (Gy)			Mean LAD dose (Gy)		
				FB	DIBH	Reduction with DIBH	FB	DIBH	Reduction with DIBH
Vikstrom et al. [75]	vDIBH (RPM)	17	Breast	3.7	1.7	54%	18.1	6.4	65%
Hayden et al. [27]	vDIBH (RPM)	30	Breast + boost	6.9	4.0	42%	33.7	21.9	35%[e]
Hjelstuen et al. [30]	vDIBH (RPM)	17	Breast + SCV + Ax + IMC LN	6.2	3.1	50%	25.0	10.9	56%
Bruzzaniti et al. [8]	vDIBH (RPM)	8	Breast	1.7	1.2	29%	9.0	2.7	70%
Lee et al. [41]	vDIBH (RPM)	25	Breast	4.5	2.5	44%	26.3	16.0	39%
Reardon et al. [55]	vDIBH (RPM)	10	Breast	1.6	0.9	45%[f]	2.5	1.8	29%[f]
Bolukbasi et al. [5]	vDIBH (RPM)	10 / 10	Breast	1.7 / 4.9	0.7 / 3.7	59%[g] / 25%[h]	1.7 / 5.0	0.8 / 4.0	53%[g] / 20%[h]
Osman et al. [51]	vDIBH (RPM)	13	Breast + SCV + Ax + IMC LN	9.0 / 5.8	5.0 / 4.1	44%[a] / 29%[b]	– / –	– / –	– / –
Verhoeven et al. [74]	vDIBH (RPM)	17	Breast	3.5	1.6	54%	30.9	22.4	28%
Joo et al. [37]	vDIBH (RPM)	32	Breast/CW ± SCV + Ax	7.2	2.8	61%	40.8	23.7	42%
Mulliez et al. [48]	vDIBH (RPM)	12	Breast	4.0	2.2	45%	17.6	10.9	38%
Rochet et al. [59]	vDIBH (other)	35	Breast/CW ± SCV + Ax + IMC LN	2.5	0.9	64%	14.9	4.0	73%

Tanguturi et al. [68]	vDIBH (AlignRT)	146	Breast/CW ± SCV + Ax ± IMC LN	2.6	1.4	46%	–	–	–
Yeung et al. [82]	vDIBH (other)	20	Breast/CW ± SCV + Ax + IMC LN	2.6	1.3	50%	13.6	4.1	70%
Walston et al. [76]	vDIBH (AlignRT)	7 / 8	Breast ± boost CW ± boost ± SCV + Ax + IMC LN	1.3 / 5.1	0.9 / 3.6	31% / 29%	– / –	– / –	– / –
Wiant et al. [80]	vDIBH (other)	25	Breast	3.0	1.4	53%	–	–	–

Abbreviations: ABC active breathing coordinator, *Ax* axillary, *CW* chest wall, *DIBH* deep inspiration breath hold, *Gy* gray, *FB* free breathing, *IMC* internal mammary chain, *LAD* left anterior descending coronary artery, *LN* lymph nodes, *RPM* real-time positioning management system, *SCV* supraclavicular

[a]3DCRT
[b]IMRT/VMAT
[c]227 left-sided (144 received DIBH; 83 received FB treatment)
[d]Median values for mean doses
[e]LAD planning risk volume (PRV)
[f]FB-IMRT versus 3D-DIBH
[g]FB versus DIBH forward-planned IMRT
[h]FB versus DIBH inverse-planned IMRT

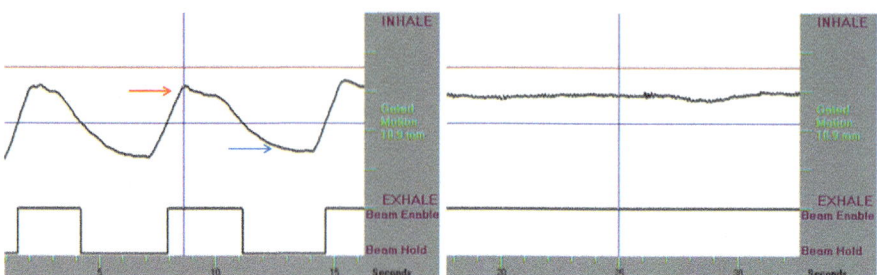

Fig. 6.4 RPM respiratory tracings verify adequate chest excursion during DIBH. The tracing on the left displays the chest wall sinusoidal excursion at inspiration (*red arrow*) and at expiration (*blue arrow*). The tracing on the right depicts a stable tracing of the same patient at deep inspiration

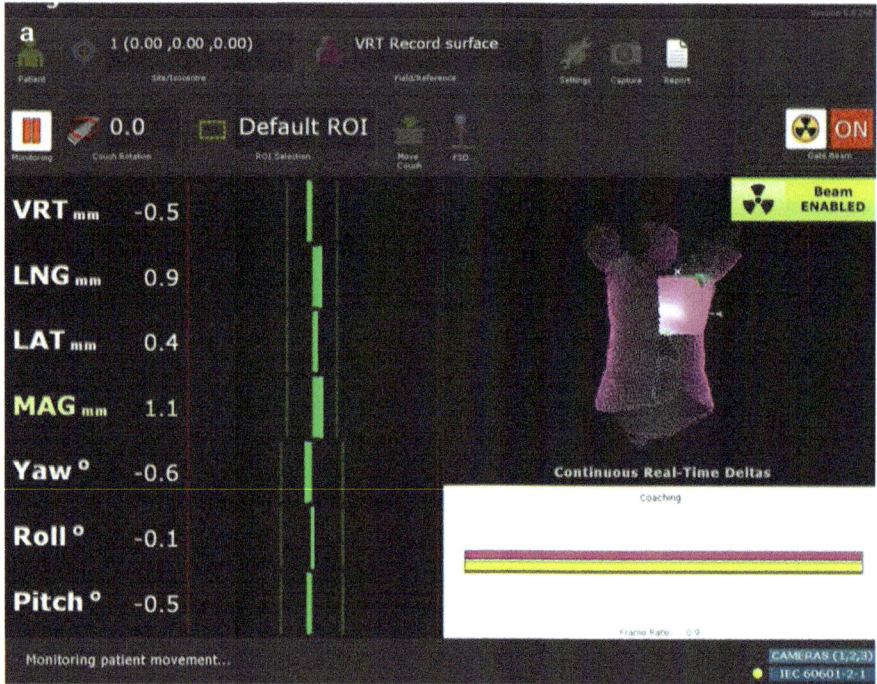

Fig 6.5 Real-time monitoring of patient voluntary breath hold accuracy using an optical tracking system. (**a**) A screenshot of AlignRT shows a reference three-dimensional surface on the right used for alignment with a region of interest (the left breast), which is matched during subsequent surface tracking. During breath hold, when the breast is within the preset thresholds (indicated by *green bars* on the left plus the coaching window at the *bottom right*) the radiation beam is enabled. (**b**) If the patient breathes out, or moves out of tolerance in any of the 6 degrees of freedom, the *green bars* on the left turn *red* and the radiation beam is automatically held. This process is repeated until the whole radiation dose has been delivered (Photo courtesy of Vision RT)

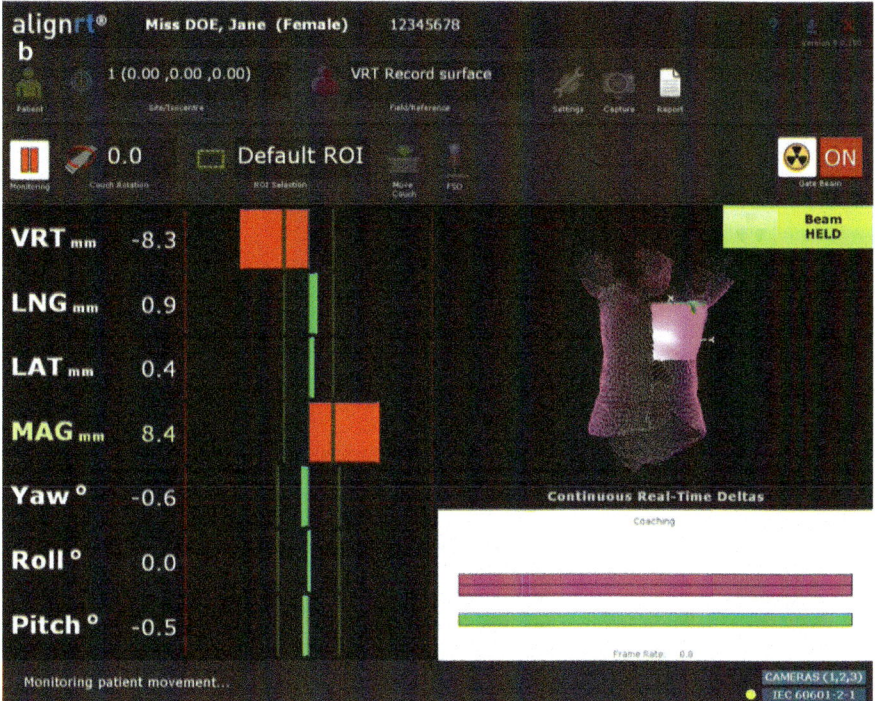

Fig 6.5 (continued)

in chest excursion for each breath within a treatment fraction and within a treatment field were very small, demonstrating reliable geometry of the chest wall [4]. Another study also showed high patient setup accuracy using optical surface imaging [69]. Similarly, when magnetic sensors were affixed to the thorax to measure chest excursion during DIBH, the standard deviation of the amplitude of chest motion comparing breaths for each patient was <3 mm, indicating that the magnitude of inspiration could be reliably reproduced [56].

For vDIBH, patients must voluntarily breathe to reach a predefined threshold or gating window. The treatment beam is stopped automatically or manually when the patient's breathing falls outside the preset threshold. In addition to the previously discussed vDIBH methods, visual monitoring of lateral tattoo positions using lasers (Fig. 6.6) [3, 35], real-time distance-measuring laser devices [35], fluoroscopy image-guided methods [6], and some combination of these techniques [44] for vDIBH have been described. Active coaching and visual patient feedback devices may also be combined with other vDIBH techniques ([41] and reviewed in Latty et al. [40]). In addition, continuous cine imaging using an electronic portal imaging device indicates the stability of the chest wall and verifies that the cardiac shadow has not entered the radiation port (Fig. 6.7).

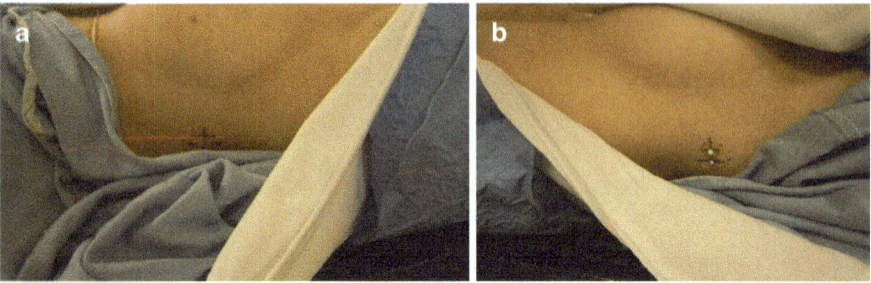

Fig. 6.6 Lateral level marks at free breathing and deep inspiration can verify accurate positioning during treatment. (**a**) A laser at the level of the lateral leveling mark at free breathing. (**b**) A large BB marker is placed over the free breathing lateral leveling mark and a small BB marker over the position of the same lasers at deep inspiration, allowing remote verification of positioning during treatment using a magnification camera

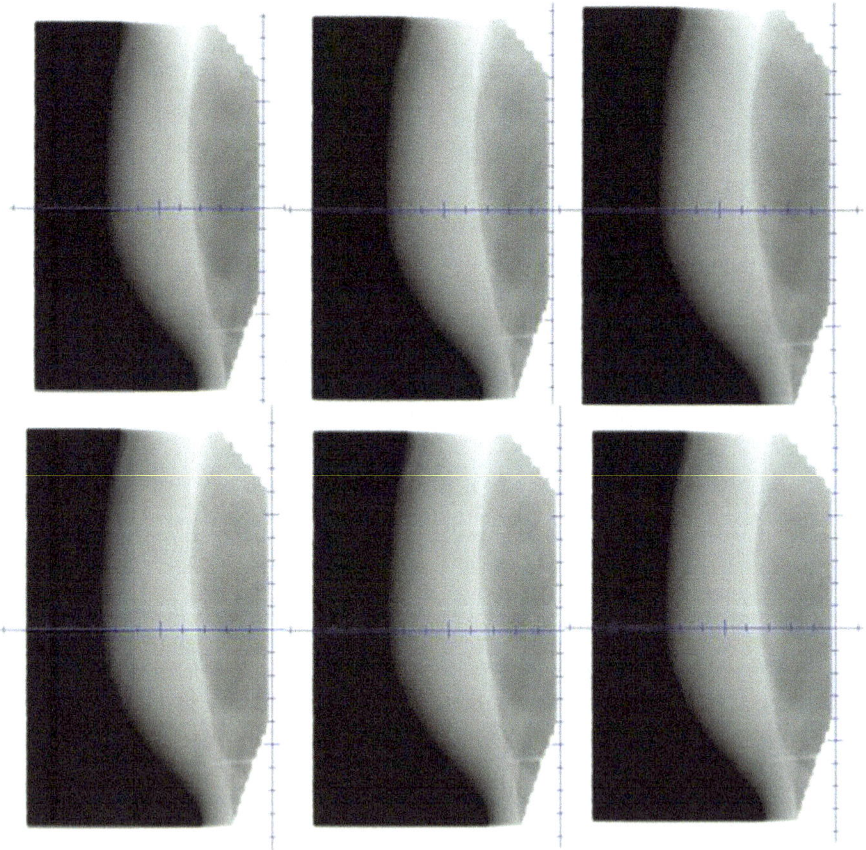

Fig. 6.7 Cine imaging indicates the stability of the chest wall and omission of the heart from the radiation field during treatment. These 6 MV films represent a capture of the treatment beam on the imager over the course of a single lateral left tangent field. They look almost identical, confirming the stability of the chest wall during deep inspiration breath hold. Note the absence of the cardiac shadow in all images

Some have questioned the necessity of ABC and thus have utilized vDIBH techniques. Several vDIBH techniques may be implemented at relatively low cost [3, 44]. The UK HeartSpare Study [3] was a randomized crossover study in which patients treated with left-sided breast cancer were randomly assigned to receive initial treatment with vDIBH or ABC. Patients received the other DIBH technique for the second half of treatment. The vDIBH method was fairly simple, visualizing skin marks using an in-room camera. Electronic portal imaging and cone beam computed tomography revealed no difference in setup variability or dose to the heart or lungs between vDIBH and ABC. While actual treatment times were comparable, setup time and simulation times were shorter with vDIBH. Surveys of patients and radiation therapists showed that both groups were more satisfied with vDIBH [3], similar to a previous report in which 21 of 112 enrolled patients (18%) could not tolerate the ABC device and were treated off study [19]. Thus, the choice of DIBH technique must balance setup and breathing reproducibility with patient convenience.

6.3   Dosimetric and Potential Functional Advantages of DIBH

Due to the long latency period of radiation-induced cardiac morbidity and mortality, there are currently no data demonstrating that DIBH definitively improves cardiac outcomes. However, the dosimetric advantages of using DIBH via ABC devices or vDIBH are dramatic, with decreases in mean doses to the heart and left anterior descending coronary artery (LAD) of 25–67% and 20–71%, respectively (Table 6.1). An example dose volume histogram showing decreases in radiation doses to the heart and LAD for a free breathing versus vDIBH 3DCRT plan appears in Fig. 6.8. DIBH leads to improvements in mean heart and LAD doses for patients treated via 3DCRT and IMRT and for patients receiving regional nodal treatment as well as breast or chest wall therapy alone (reviewed in [64]).

Perfusion defects have been detected in patients who received left-sided radiation therapy; these defects corresponded with the radiation treatment fields [21, 24]. Two prospective studies that used DIBH and excluded the entire heart from the radiation beams found no myocardial perfusion defects [10, 83]. This suggests that DIBH, as part of a comprehensive strategy for reducing cardiac doses of radiation, may incrementally reduce cardiac damage. In contrast, a small randomized trial that compared ABC DIBH with free breathing found that the incidence of myocardial perfusion defects did not differ between the treatment arms [84]. This study did not require the heart to be excluded from the radiotherapy beams. It is not clear how to reconcile these disparate conclusions. Perhaps the lesson is that the cardiac dose of radiation must be kept very low in order to prevent perfusion changes. Taken together, the available data suggest that the use of DIBH techniques to decrease heart radiation exposure has the potential to decrease the risk of radiation-induced cardiac morbidity [19].

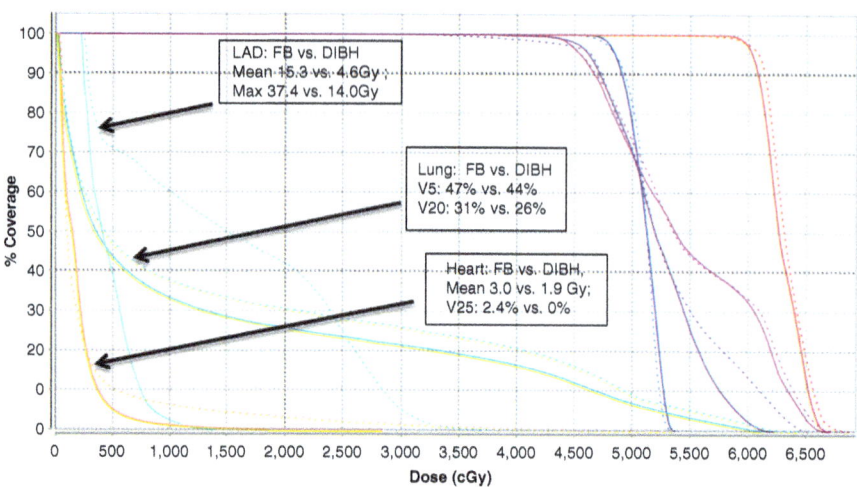

Fig. 6.8 Example of a dose volume histogram comparison of free breathing and DIBH plans. Both the free breathing and DIBH plan for this patient treated the left chest wall to 50 Gy plus a 10 Gy boost and regional lymph nodes including the supraclavicular and IMC nodes. The organs at risk in the DIBH plan (*solid lines*), including the heart (*orange lines*), left lung (*green lines*), and LAD (*light blue lines*), demonstrated decreased radiation doses when compared to the free breathing plan (*dotted lines*)

6.4 Patient Selection and Treatment Planning

Many DIBH techniques are relatively straightforward and well-tolerated. However, for reasons of cost, convenience, and throughput, it may be necessary to select patients for DIBH on the basis of projected benefit. Several clinical variables identify the patients most likely to benefit from DIBH; the most obvious selection criterion is cancer laterality. The heart sits to the left side of the thoracic cavity and heart dose is higher for patients treated to the left breast/chest wall than to the right. This dosimetric difference translates to a meaningful clinical difference in outcomes: the risk of cardiac mortality is higher after left breast irradiation [15]. Therefore, most institutions limit DIBH to left-sided breast cancers. Although DIBH reduces the cardiac dose to women receiving radiotherapy to the breast without nodal coverage, the magnitude of reduction in heart dose is larger for women receiving radiotherapy to the IMC as well [82]. Therefore, it is most important to consider using DIBH in patients receiving radiotherapy to the left breast/chest wall and the IMC.

Individual anatomical data may also predict the benefit of DIBH. Maximal heart distance (measured as the maximal distance between the anterior cardiac contour and the posterior tangential field edges) is strongly correlated with heart dose [38, 71]. Similarly, parasagittal cardiac contact distance is associated with several cardiac dose parameters for women undergoing free breathing as well as DIBH [59]. Thus, maximal heart distance and/or parasagittal cardiac contact distance could be measured at the time of free breathing computed tomography simulation and then used as selection criteria for rescanning the patient at DIBH. Computed tomography carried out during free breathing and DIBH can be compared without creating two complete treatment plans. The benefit of DIBH over free breathing is correlated to the change in lung volume between the two scans: patients that experienced the largest change in lung volume between scans achieved the largest reduction in heart dose [68]. On the other hand, at least three-quarters of women derive a meaningful benefit from DIBH [59], supporting the routine use of DIBH for most women with left-sided breast cancer.

It is our current preference that all women treated with radiotherapy to the left breast or chest wall in the supine position undergo computed tomography during both free breathing and DIBH. The radiation oncologist should review both scans and select the optimal scan for contouring and planning based on observed cardiac motion as well as patient comfort with DIBH. In our experience, the vast majority of left-sided breast cancer patients derive sufficient benefit to merit the use of DIBH. However, this strategy requires an investment in resources. In resource-limited environments, the use of one or more of the above strategies for patient selection may be warranted. A less resource-intensive approach is to use a heart block on the tangential fields. In the breast-conserving setting, a heart block may be considered as an alternative to DIBH, depending on the location of the tumor bed in relation to the block. We typically do not use this technique in the mastectomy setting if it results in blocking of the ipsilateral chest wall.

Once the decision for DIBH has been made, treatment planning begins. Several dosimetric analyses are available for free breathing patients that compare three-dimensional conformal beam arrangements as well as IMRT [33, 53, 72]. More complex photon-electron matched plans have also been described [50]. Although no beam arrangement is optimal for all patients, multiple reports favor partially wide tangents over other three-dimensional conformal techniques to include the IMC [53, 72]. The partially wide tangent technique delivers even lower cardiac doses when paired with DIBH [66]. Overall, planning decisions for DIBH and free breathing are similar. Treatment delivery techniques for DIBH include 3DCRT, IMRT, and volumetric arc therapy [5, 51, 66].

It is important to consider the multiple sources of intra- and interfraction uncertainty when contouring targets and normal structures. Reassuringly, the interfraction positional variability of the LAD is comparable between DIBH and free breathing [34]. Similarly, analyses of the interfraction and intrafraction motion of the breast at DIBH indicate impressive stability and reproducibility of breast position [4, 23], particularly with bony anatomy (typical shifts of 0.1–0.2 cm in each axis [46]). However, the LAD, perhaps the most important target for radiotherapy-induced heart disease from tangential breast irradiation, exhibits some variability in its displacement on DIBH [78]. Even if this geometric variability averages out (if the average of daily setup errors are nondirectional), it may translate into the delivery of consistently higher cardiac doses than predicted at planning because the steep dose gradient at the field edge could yield a dramatic increase in heart dose when a field sets up "deep" but a small decrease in heart dose when a field is "shallow." For these reasons, a planning organ at risk volume (PRV) expansion of 0.5 cm around the LAD has been proposed [78].

When starting a new DIBH program, we suggest a stepwise progression of treatment complexity, starting with irradiation of the breast alone using tangential fields prior to incorporating more complex techniques necessary for irradiating regional nodes. It may also be helpful for patient compliance to minimize the time of delivery of each beam. We suggest limiting the number of beam segments per field and maximizing the dose rate of the linear accelerator in order to keep the total time of beam delivery relatively short. With regard to contouring and cardiac sparing, we suggest that the field edge be spaced a few millimeters from the cardiac shadow if possible, in order to exclude the heart from the radiotherapy beams even with small variations in setup.

Conclusions

Radiotherapy is a valuable adjuvant treatment in breast cancer that improves locoregional control and overall survival. New data show that in selected patients, the inclusion of regional nodal basins in the radiotherapy field incrementally reduces the risk of recurrence versus breast radiotherapy alone. However, breast radiotherapy inevitably delivers some radiation to the heart. The treatment of left-sided breast cancer and the inclusion of the IMC are associated with higher average cardiac doses. In the short term, cardiac irradiation can lead to perfusion changes in the radiation field. Over the long term, radiotherapy is associated with a dose-dependent elevation in the risk of cardiac morbidity and mortality, motivating the minimization of cardiac dose.

DIBH expands the lungs and moves the heart away from the breast during radiotherapy. DIBH can be accomplished through a variety of techniques, some of which are relatively simple to implement and inexpensive. Multiple studies have reported that DIBH yields inter- and intrafraction reproducibility equivalent to those of free breathing. DIBH unambiguously reduces cardiac dose in dosimetric analyses, and early clinical data suggest that this reduction in cardiac dose translates into avoidance of the expected changes in cardiac perfusion. Although additional clinical data are required, DIBH offers the tantalizing potential of maintaining the benefits of radiotherapy while minimizing cardiac risks. Further research aimed to refine techniques and to optimize patient selection is ongoing.

References

1. Alderliesten T, Sonke J-J, Betgen A et al (2013) Accuracy evaluation of a 3-dimensional surface imaging system for guidance in deep-inspiration breath-hold radiation therapy. Int J Radiat Oncol Biol Phys 85:536–542
2. Ares C, Khan S, MacArtain AM et al (2010) Postoperative proton radiotherapy for localized and locoregional breast cancer: potential for clinically relevant improvements? Int J Radiat Oncol Biol Phys 76:685–697

3. Bartlett FR, Colgan RM, Carr K et al (2013) The UK HeartSpare Study: randomised evaluation of voluntary deep-inspiratory breath-hold in women undergoing breast radiotherapy. Radiother Oncol 108:242–247

4. Betgen A, Alderliesten T, Sonke J-J et al (2013) Assessment of set-up variability during deep inspiration breath hold radiotherapy for breast cancer patients by 3D-surface imaging. Radiother Oncol 106:225–230

5. Bolukbasi Y, Saglam Y, Selek U et al (2014) Reproducible deep-inspiration breath-hold irradiation with forward intensity-modulated radiotherapy for left-sided breast cancer significantly reduces cardiac radiation exposure compared to inverse intensity-modulated radiotherapy. Tumori 100:169–178

6. Borst GR, Sonke J-J, den Hollander S et al (2010) Clinical results of image-guided deep inspiration breath hold breast irradiation. Int J Radiat Oncol Biol Phys 78:1345–1351

7. Bouillon K, Haddy N, Delaloge S et al (2011) Long-term cardiovascular mortality after radiotherapy for breast cancer. J Am Coll Cardiol 57:445–452

8. Bruzzaniti V, Abate A, Pinnarò P et al (2013) Dosimetric and clinical advantages of deep inspiration breath-hold (DIBH) during radiotherapy of breast cancer. J Exp Clin Cancer Res CR 32:88

9. Chargari C, Castadot P, Macdermed D et al (2010) Internal mammary lymph node irradiation contributes to heart dose in breast cancer. Med Dosim 35:163–168

10. Chung E, Corbett JR, Moran JM et al (2013) Is there a dose-response relationship for heart disease with low-dose radiation therapy? Int J Radiat Oncol Biol Phys 85:959–964

11. Clarke M, Collins R, Darby S et al (2005) Effects of radiotherapy and of differences in the extent of surgery for early breast cancer on local recurrence and 15-year survival: an overview of the randomised trials. Lancet 366:2087–2106

12. Comsa D, Barnett E, Le K et al (2014) Introduction of moderate deep inspiration breath hold for radiation therapy of left breast: Initial experience of a regional cancer center. Pract Radiat Oncol 4:298–305

13. Cuzick J, Stewart H, Rutqvist L et al (1994) Cause-specific mortality in long-term survivors of breast cancer who participated in trials of radiotherapy. J Clin Oncol 12:447–453

14. Darby SC, Ewertz M, McGale P et al (2013) Risk of ischemic heart disease in women after radiotherapy for breast cancer. N Engl J Med 368:987–998

15. Darby SC, McGale P, Taylor CW, Peto R (2005) Long-term mortality from heart disease and lung cancer after radiotherapy for early breast cancer: prospective cohort study of about 300,000 women in US SEER cancer registries. Lancet Oncol 6:557–565

16. Early Breast Cancer Trialists' Collaborative Group (EBCTCG) (2000) Favourable and unfavourable effects on long-term survival of radiotherapy for early breast cancer: an overview of the randomised trials. Lancet 355:1757–1770

17. Early Breast Cancer Trialists' Collaborative Group (EBCTCG), Darby S, McGale P et al (2011) Effect of radiotherapy after breast-conserving surgery on 10-year recurrence and 15-year breast cancer death: meta-analysis of individual patient data for 10,801 women in 17 randomised trials. Lancet 378:1707–1716

18. Early Breast Cancer Trialists' Collaborative Group (EBCTCG), McGale P, Taylor C et al (2014) Effect of radiotherapy after mastectomy and axillary surgery on 10-year recurrence and 20-year breast cancer mortality: meta-analysis of individual patient data for 8135 women in 22 randomised trials. Lancet 383:2127–2135

19. Eldredge-Hindy HB, Duffy D, Yamoah K et al (2015) Modeled risk of ischemic heart disease following left breast irradiation with deep inspiration breath hold. Pract Radiat Oncol 5:162–168

20. Eldredge-Hindy H, Lockamy V, Crawford A et al (2015) Active breathing coordinator reduces radiation dose to the heart and preserves local control in patients with left breast cancer: report of a prospective trial. Pract Radiat Oncol 5:4–10

21. Evans ES, Prosnitz RG, Yu X et al (2006) Impact of patient-specific factors, irradiated left ventricular volume, and treatment set-up errors on the development of myocardial perfu-

sion defects after radiation therapy for left-sided breast cancer. Int J Radiat Oncol Biol Phys 66:1125–1134

22. Formenti SC, DeWyngaert J, Jozsef G, Goldberg JD (2012) Prone vs supine positioning for breast cancer radiotherapy. JAMA 308:861–863

23. Gierga DP, Turcotte JC, Sharp GC et al (2012) A voluntary breath-hold treatment technique for the left breast with unfavorable cardiac anatomy using surface imaging. Int J Radiat Oncol Biol Phys 84:e663–e668

24. Gyenes G, Fornander T, Carlens P et al (1997) Detection of radiation-induced myocardial damage by technetium-99m sestamibi scintigraphy. Eur J Nucl Med 24:286–292

25. Gyenes G, Rutqvist LE, Liedberg A, Fornander T (1998) Long-term cardiac morbidity and mortality in a randomized trial of pre- and postoperative radiation therapy versus surgery alone in primary breast cancer. Radiother Oncol 48:185–190

26. Harris EER, Correa C, Hwang W-T et al (2006) Late cardiac mortality and morbidity in early-stage breast cancer patients after breast-conservation treatment. J Clin Oncol 24:4100–4106

27. Hayden AJ, Rains M, Tiver K (2012) Deep inspiration breath hold technique reduces heart dose from radiotherapy for left-sided breast cancer. J Med Imaging Radiat Oncol 56:464–472

28. Hennequin C, Bossard N, Servagi-Vernat S et al (2013) Ten-year survival results of a randomized trial of irradiation of internal mammary nodes after mastectomy. Int J Radiat Oncol Biol Phys 86:860–866

29. Henson KE, McGale P, Taylor C, Darby SC (2013) Radiation-related mortality from heart disease and lung cancer more than 20 years after radiotherapy for breast cancer. Br J Cancer 108:179–182

30. Hjelstuen MHB, Mjaaland I, Vikström J, Dybvik KI (2012) Radiation during deep inspiration allows loco-regional treatment of left breast and axillary-, supraclavicular- and internal mammary lymph nodes without compromising target coverage or dose restrictions to organs at risk. Acta Oncol 51:333–344

31. Hooning MJ, Aleman BMP, van Rosmalen AJM et al (2006) Cause-specific mortality in long-term survivors of breast cancer: a 25-year follow-up study. Int J Radiat Oncol 64:1081–1091

32. Hooning MJ, Botma A, Aleman BMP et al (2007) Long-term risk of cardiovascular disease in 10-year survivors of breast cancer. J Natl Cancer Inst 99:365–375

33. Jagsi R, Moran J, Marsh R et al (2010) Evaluation of four techniques using intensity-modulated radiation therapy for comprehensive locoregional irradiation of breast cancer. Int J Radiat Oncol Biol Phys 78:1594–1603

34. Jagsi R, Moran JM, Kessler ML et al (2007) Respiratory motion of the heart and positional reproducibility under active breathing control. Int J Radiat Oncol Biol Phys 68:253–258

35. Jensen C, Urribarri J, Cail D et al (2014) Cine EPID evaluation of two non-commercial techniques for DIBH. Med Phys 41:021730

36. Johansen S, Vikström J, Hjelstuen MHB et al (2011) Dose evaluation and risk estimation for secondary cancer in contralateral breast and a study of correlation between thorax shape and dose to organs at risk following tangentially breast irradiation during deep inspiration breath-hold and free breathing. Acta Oncol 50:563–568

37. Joo JH, Kim SS, Ahn SD et al (2015) Cardiac dose reduction during tangential breast irradiation using deep inspiration breath hold: a dose comparison study based on deformable image registration. Radiat Oncol 10:264

38. Kong F-M, Klein EE, Bradley JD et al (2002) The impact of central lung distance, maximal heart distance, and radiation technique on the volumetric dose of the lung and heart for intact breast radiation. Int J Radiat Oncol Biol Phys 54:963–971

39. Kubo HD, Len PM, Minohara S, Mostafavi H (2000) Breathing-synchronized radiotherapy program at the University of California Davis Cancer Center. Med Phys 27:346–353

40. Latty D, Stuart KE, Wang W, Ahern V (2015) Review of deep inspiration breath-hold techniques for the treatment of breast cancer. J Med Radiat Sci 62:74–81

41. Lee HY, Chang JS, Lee IJ et al (2013) The deep inspiration breath hold technique using Abches reduces cardiac dose in patients undergoing left-sided breast irradiation. Radiat Oncol J 31:239–246

42. Lohr F, El-Haddad M, Dobler B et al (2009) Potential effect of robust and simple IMRT approach for left-sided breast cancer on cardiac mortality. Int J Radiat Oncol Biol Phys 74:73–80

43. MacDonald SM, Jimenez R, Paetzold P et al (2013) Proton radiotherapy for chest wall and regional lymphatic radiation; dose comparisons and treatment delivery. Radiat Oncol 8:71

44. Macrie BD, Donnelly ED, Hayes JP et al (2015) A cost-effective technique for cardiac sparing with deep inspiration-breath hold (DIBH). Phys Medica 31:733–737

45. Mast ME, van Kempen-Harteveld L, Heijenbrok MW et al (2013) Left-sided breast cancer radiotherapy with and without breath-hold: does IMRT reduce the cardiac dose even further? Radiother Oncol 108:248–253

46. McIntosh A, Shoushtari AN, Benedict SH et al (2011) Quantifying the reproducibility of heart position during treatment and corresponding delivered heart dose in voluntary deep inhalation breath hold for left breast cancer patients treated with external beam radiotherapy. Int J Radiat Oncol Biol Phys 81:e569–e576

47. Mulliez T, Van de Velde J, Veldeman L et al (2015) Deep inspiration breath hold in the prone position retracts the heart from the breast and internal mammary lymph node region. Radiother Oncol 117:473–476

48. Mulliez T, Veldeman L, Speleers B et al (2015) Heart dose reduction by prone deep inspiration breath hold in left-sided breast irradiation. Radiother Oncol 114:79–84

49. Nissen HD, Appelt AL (2013) Improved heart, lung and target dose with deep inspiration breath hold in a large clinical series of breast cancer patients. Radiother Oncol 106:28–32

50. Oh JL, Buchholz TA (2009) Internal mammary node radiation: a proposed technique to spare cardiac toxicity. J Clin Oncol 27:e172–e173

51. Osman SOS, Hol S, Poortmans PM, Essers M (2014) Volumetric modulated arc therapy and breath-hold in image-guided locoregional left-sided breast irradiation. Radiother Oncol 112:17–22

52. Peng JL, Kahler D, Li JG et al (2010) Characterization of a real-time surface image-guided stereotactic positioning system. Med Phys 37:5421–5433

53. Pierce LJ, Butler JB, Martel MK et al (2002) Postmastectomy radiotherapy of the chest wall: dosimetric comparison of common techniques. Int J Radiat Oncol Biol Phys 52:1220–1230

54. Poortmans PM, Collette S, Kirkove C et al (2015) Internal mammary and medial supraclavicular irradiation in breast cancer. N Engl J Med 373:317–327

55. Reardon KA, Read PW, Morris MM et al (2013) A comparative analysis of 3D conformal deep inspiratory-breath hold and free-breathing intensity-modulated radiation therapy for left-sided breast cancer. Med Dosim 38:190–195

56. Remouchamps VM, Huyskens DP, Mertens I et al (2007) The use of magnetic sensors to monitor moderate deep inspiration breath hold during breast irradiation with dynamic MLC compensators. Radiother Oncol 82:341–348

57. Remouchamps VM, Letts N, Vicini FA et al (2003) Initial clinical experience with moderate deep-inspiration breath hold using an active breathing control device in the treatment of patients with left-sided breast cancer using external beam radiation therapy. Int J Radiat Oncol Biol Phys 56:704–715

58. Remouchamps VM, Vicini FA, Sharpe MB et al (2003) Significant reductions in heart and lung doses using deep inspiration breath hold with active breathing control and intensity-modulated radiation therapy for patients treated with locoregional breast irradiation. Int J Radiat Oncol Biol Phys 55:392–406

59. Rochet N, Drake JI, Harrington K et al (2015) Deep inspiration breath-hold technique in left-sided breast cancer radiation therapy: evaluating cardiac contact distance as a predictor of cardiac exposure for patient selection. Pract Radiat Oncol 5:e127–e134

60. Rong Y, Walston S, Welliver MX et al (2014) Improving intra-fractional target position accuracy using a 3D surface surrogate for left breast irradiation using the respiratory-gated deep-inspiration breath-hold technique. PLoS One 9(5):e97933

61. Rutqvist LE, Johansson H (1990) Mortality by laterality of the primary tumour among 55,000 breast cancer patients from the Swedish Cancer Registry. Br J Cancer 61:866–868

62. Sardaro A, Petruzzelli MF, D'Errico MP et al (2012) Radiation-induced cardiac damage in early left breast cancer patients: risk factors, biological mechanisms, radiobiology, and dosimetric constraints. Radiother Oncol 103:133–142
63. Shapiro CL, Hardenbergh PH, Gelman R et al (1998) Cardiac effects of adjuvant doxorubicin and radiation therapy in breast cancer patients. J Clin Oncol 16:3493–3501
64. Smyth LM, Knight KA, Aarons YK, Wasiak J (2015) The cardiac dose-sparing benefits of deep inspiration breath-hold in left breast irradiation: a systematic review. J Med Radiat Sci 62:66–73
65. Stranzl H, Zurl B (2008) Postoperative irradiation of left-sided breast cancer patients and cardiac toxicity. Does deep inspiration breath-hold (DIBH) technique protect the heart? Strahlenther Onkol 184:354–358
66. Stranzl H, Zurl B, Langsenlehner T, Kapp KS (2009) Wide tangential fields including the internal mammary lymph nodes in patients with left-sided breast cancer. Influence of respiratory-controlled radiotherapy (4D-CT) on cardiac exposure. Strahlenther Onkol 185:155–160
67. Swanson T, Grills IS, Ye H et al (2013) Six-year experience routinely using moderate deep inspiration breath-hold for the reduction of cardiac dose in left-sided breast irradiation for patients with early-stage or locally advanced breast cancer. Am J Clin Oncol 36:24–30
68. Tanguturi SK, Lyatskaya Y, Chen Y et al (2015) Prospective assessment of deep inspiration breath-hold using 3-dimensional surface tracking for irradiation of left-sided breast cancer. Pract Radiat Oncol 5:358–365
69. Tang X, Zagar TM, Bair E et al (2014) Clinical experience with 3-dimensional surface matching-based deep inspiration breath hold for left-sided breast cancer radiation therapy. Pract Radiat Oncol 4:e151–e158
70. Taylor C, Correa C, Anderson S et al (2015) Late side-effects of breast cancer radiotherapy: Second incidence and non-breast-cancer mortality among 40,000 women in 75 trials. San Antonio Breast Cancer Symp S5:08(Abstract)
71. Taylor CW, McGale P, Povall JM et al (2009) Estimating cardiac exposure from breast cancer radiotherapy in clinical practice. Int J Radiat Oncol Biol Phys 73:1061–1068
72. Thomsen MS, Berg M, Nielsen HM et al (2008) Post-mastectomy radiotherapy in Denmark: from 2D to 3D treatment planning guidelines of The Danish Breast Cancer Cooperative Group. Acta Oncol 47:654–661
73. Thorsen LBJ, Offersen BV, Danø H et al (2016) DBCG-IMN: a population-based cohort study on the effect of internal mammary node irradiation in early node-positive breast cancer. J Clin Oncol 34:314–320
74. Verhoeven K, Sweldens C, Petillion S et al (2014) Breathing adapted radiation therapy in comparison with prone position to reduce the doses to the heart, left anterior descending coronary artery, and contralateral breast in whole breast radiation therapy. Pract Radiat Oncol 4:123–129
75. Vikström J, Hjelstuen MHB, Mjaaland I, Dybvik KI (2011) Cardiac and pulmonary dose reduction for tangentially irradiated breast cancer, utilizing deep inspiration breath-hold with audio-visual guidance, without compromising target coverage. Acta Oncol 50:42–50
76. Walston S, Quick AM, Kuhn K, Rong Y (2016) Dosimetric considerations in respiratory-gated deep inspiration breath-hold for left breast irradiation. Technol Cancer Res Treat [Epub 2016]. doi: 10.1177/1533034615624311
77. Wang W, Purdie TG, Rahman M et al (2012) Rapid automated treatment planning process to select breast cancer patients for active breathing control to achieve cardiac dose reduction. Int J Radiat Oncol Biol Phys 82:386–393
78. Wang X, Pan T, Pinnix C et al (2012) Cardiac motion during deep-inspiration breath-hold: implications for breast cancer radiotherapy. Int J Radiat Oncol Biol Phys 82:708–714
79. Whelan TJ, Olivotto IA, Parulekar WR et al (2015) Regional nodal irradiation in early-stage breast cancer. N Engl J Med 373:307–316

80. Wiant D, Wentworth S, Liu H, Sintay B (2015) How important is a reproducible breath hold for deep inspiration breath hold breast radiation therapy? Int J Radiat Oncol Biol Phys 93:901–907
81. Wong JW, Sharpe MB, Jaffray DA et al (1999) The use of active breathing control (ABC) to reduce margin for breathing motion. Int J Radiat Oncol Biol Phys 44:911–919
82. Yeung R, Conroy L, Long K et al (2015) Cardiac dose reduction with deep inspiration breath hold for left-sided breast cancer radiotherapy patients with and without regional nodal irradiation. Radiat Oncol 10:200
83. Zagar TM, Tang X, Jones EL et al (2015) Prospective assessment of deep inspiration breath hold to prevent radiation associated cardiac perfusion defects in patients with left-sided breast cancer. Int J Radiat Oncol Biol Phys 93, E11
84. Zellars R, Bravo PE, Tryggestad E et al (2014) SPECT analysis of cardiac perfusion changes after whole-breast/chest wall radiation therapy with or without active breathing coordinator: results of a randomized phase 3 trial. Int J Radiat Oncol Biol Phys 88:778–785

Intensity-Modulated Radiation Therapy for Breast Cancer

7

Vishruta Dumane, Licheng Kuo, Linda Hong, and Alice Y. Ho

Contents

V. Dumane, PhD
Department of Radiation Oncology, Icahn School of Medicine at Mount Sinai, New York, NY 10029, USA

L. Kuo, MSc • L. Hong, PhD, DABR
Department of Medical Physics, Memorial Sloan Kettering Cancer Center, 1275 York Avenue, New York, NY 10065, USA

A.Y. Ho, MD (⊠)
Department of Radiation Oncology, Memorial Sloan Kettering Cancer Center, New York, NY, USA
e-mail: HoA1234@mskcc.org

© Springer International Publishing Switzerland 2016
J.R. Bellon et al. (eds.), *Radiation Therapy Techniques and Treatment Planning for Breast Cancer*, Practical Guides in Radiation Oncology,
DOI 10.1007/978-3-319-40392-2_7

7.1   Introduction

Radiotherapy is a key component of breast conservation therapy and serves an important role as adjuvant therapy after mastectomy in select node-positive breast cancer. Over the past decade, many different modalities of radiotherapy delivery have evolved, with the common goal of improving target volume coverage while minimizing high radiation doses to the adjacent normal organs. One method of radiation delivery that has been increasingly utilized as a planning tool is intensity-modulated radiotherapy (IMRT).

In contrast to three-dimensional (3D) conformal radiation therapy, which uses 2–5 static beams and wedges, intensity-modulated radiation therapy (IMRT) modulates the beam profile and aims to produce a uniform dose distribution within the treated volume of the breast/chest wall while optimally sparing the adjacent critical organs. Randomized trials as well as studies performing dosimetric comparisons of IMRT vs. 3D conformal radiation in breast-conserved patients showed that tangential IMRT improves dose homogeneity in the breast and lowers dose to the contralateral breast and the heart [1–15]. These dosimetric gains have translated into a lower risk of acute skin toxicity [9] and improved long-term cosmetic outcome compared to patients treated with conventional techniques [10, 11].

In this chapter, we will discuss different types of IMRT delivery for breast cancer, with respect to the number of beams, their arrangement, and type of optimization (inverse planning versus forward planning). We will also discuss a special type of IMRT called volumetric modulated arc therapy (VMAT) and describe its dosimetry and treatment delivery. The cumulative benefits of using VMAT in combination with breath-hold techniques to help reduce cardiac doses for left-sided breast cancer will also be addressed followed by a section on simulation and setup verification for IMRT.

7.2   Tangential IMRT for the Whole Breast

When the goal of treatment is to only treat the whole breast, IMRT can be delivered using tangential fields with either inverse or forward planning. In inverse planning, the treatment planner specifies the desired dose distribution and constraints to an optimization algorithm. There is hence a need to contour a planning target volume (PTV) and organs at risk (OARs) to be spared, so that this information can be used by the algorithm/optimization engine to generate the optimal beam intensity profile for each tangential beam. Forward planning, however, does not use such an algorithm and therefore does not require the definition of a PTV and OARs. Beam intensity profiles are designed by combining multiple MLC (multi-leaf collimator) segments, which are constructed from isodose distributions produced by an open tangential field plan. This is also referred to as field-in-field technique. Both inverse and forward planning techniques have demonstrated significant improvements in dose homogeneity as well as in sparing of critical organs compared to conventional techniques [12–15].

Fig. 7.1 Contours for a tangential field IMRT plan. Indicated are the PTV, heart, left ventricle, contralateral breast, ipsilateral lung, and contralateral lung

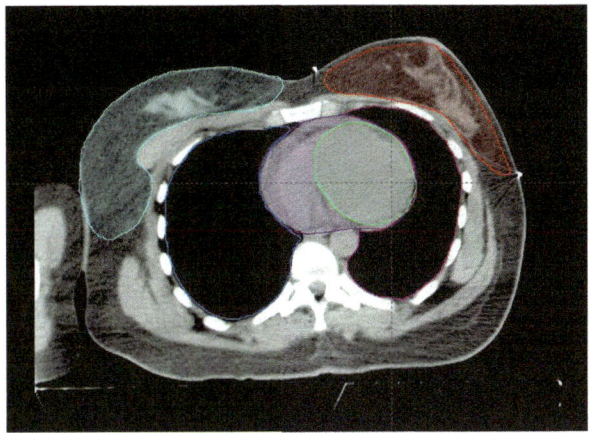

7.2.1   Whole Breast IMRT with Inverse Planning

Whole breast IMRT with inverse planning was the first IMRT technique to be applied for treating the intact breast without any nodal involvement and was developed at Memorial Sloan-Kettering Cancer Center in 1999 [14]. The field arrangement is identical to that used for a standard 3D conformal plan, consisting of two tangential beams. The physician contours the PTV and the OARs, which include the ipsilateral lung, contralateral lung, contralateral breast, heart, and left ventricle as shown in Fig. 7.1. The planner defines the prescription dose and dose homogeneity objectives for the PTV, along with dose-volume objectives for the OARs in the optimization engine. Each objective has an associated penalty, which indicates to the optimizer how hard it has to work in order to achieve the objective. The output of this algorithm is an optimal fluence for each tangential beam as indicated in Fig. 7.2a, b. The fluence/beam intensity profile is nonuniform for each beam, compared to a standard wedge profile, due to the compensation for variation in the contour of the breast as well as in its separation at different locations. The profiles of both these beams are such that a combination of their resultant dose distribution within the PTV is uniform while optimally sparing organs in the surrounding region. To account for motion due to breathing and potential swelling of the breast during the course of treatment, skin flash is added by extending the fluence beyond the skin surface by at least 2 cm. Delivery of the fluence can be accomplished in two ways, namely, dynamic multi-leaf collimator (DMLC) or multiple static field multi-leaf collimator (MSF-MLC), also referred to as step-and-shoot (SAS) delivery. In DMLC mode, the MLC moves continuously while the radiation beam is "on." In SAS mode, the MLC moves in a sequence of a discrete number of fixed-aperture shapes, and the radiation is delivered only when the MLC reaches each shape.

Comparison of the dose distribution of inverse-planned tangential field IMRT versus conventional 3D conformal planning using tangents with wedges is shown in Fig. 7.3a. Compared with the 3D plan, the IMRT plan is more homogeneous with reduced hotspots. Sparing of the critical organs was comparable between the two

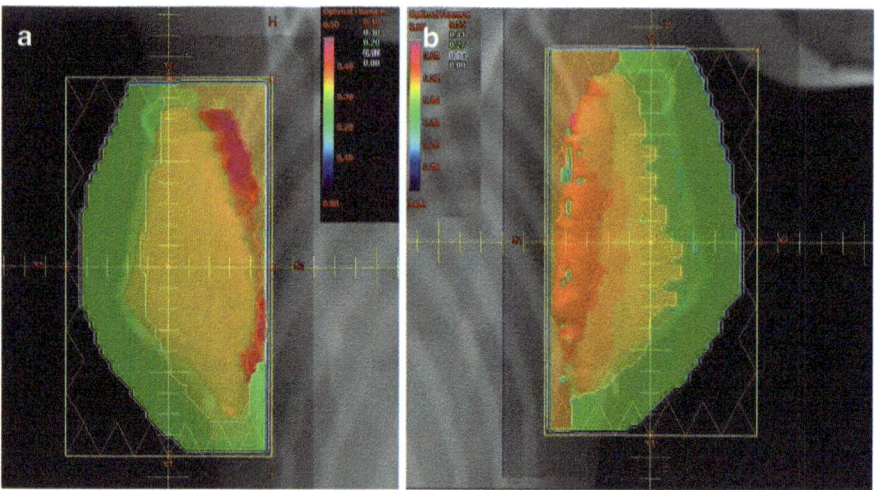

Fig. 7.2 (**a**) Optimal fluence profile of the lateral tangential beam for a left-sided intact breast case treated with tangential field IMRT. The fluence is color coded with warmer (*red*) colors indicating higher intensity levels. (**b**) Optimal fluence profile of the medial tangential beam for a left-sided intact breast case treated with tangential field IMRT

techniques. A comparison of the DVHs (dose-volume histograms) is shown in Fig. 7.3b, c. Coverage to the PTV is more homogeneous with IMRT compared to 3D planning. Because of the use of tangential fields, all dose levels, including the low dose, are confined to these fields preventing its spread to underlying ipsilateral as well as contralateral structures. Moreover, with the ability of inverse-planned IMRT to optimize and spare doses to critical organs, the low dose to the ipsilateral lung can be even lower than that achieved with conventional 3D conformal planning, as is shown for this case in Fig. 7.3c.

7.2.2 Whole Breast IMRT with Forward Planning

The forward IMRT planning technique, also referred to as field-in-field planning, was developed more than a decade ago [15] at the William Beaumont Hospital in order to improve dose uniformity and potentially reduce acute skin toxicity with tangential whole breast radiotherapy. A multicenter randomized trial by Pignol et al. has proven this technique to be effective in reducing acute radiation dermatitis and in improving the quality of life compared to standard methods [9]. This trial compared two treatment arms, namely, planning with wedges versus forward-planned IMRT. CT scans were acquired in all cases. In the standard arm, tungsten wedges of fixed angles were used to compensate for missing tissue and variability in the breast separation. Selection of the optimal wedge angle was done iteratively by reducing hotspots to the whole breast as calculated in 3D on the acquired CT scans. In the forward-planned IMRT arm, multiple subfields or "field in fields" were

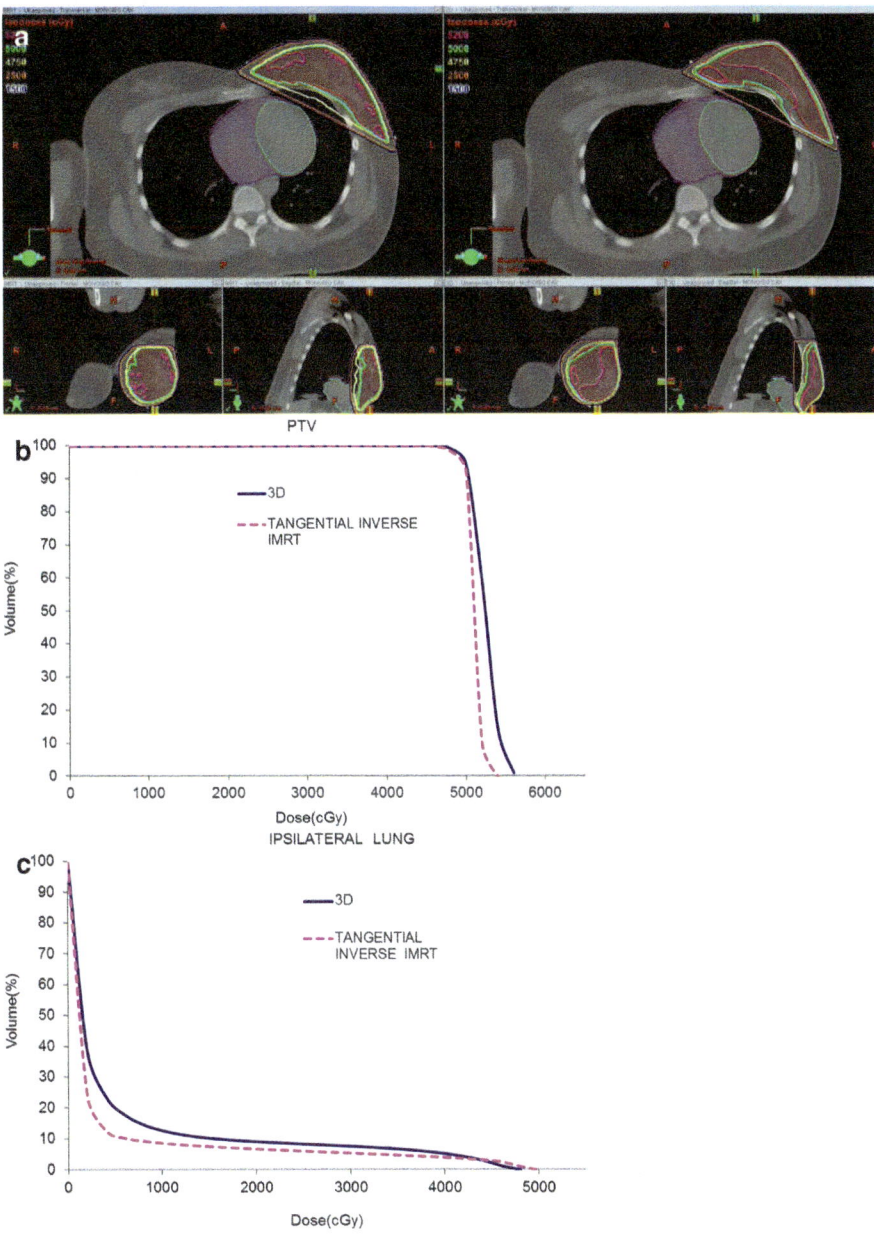

Fig. 7.3 (**a**) Dose distribution for a left-sided intact breast in the axial, coronal, and sagittal planes using tangential field inverse-planned IMRT on the left versus a standard wedge plan with tangents on the right. (**b**) Dose-volume histogram (DVH) comparing PTV coverage for the case in (**a**) with 3D versus tangential field IMRT. (**c**) Dose-volume histogram (DVH) comparing dose to the ipsilateral lung for the case in (**a**) with 3D versus tangential field IMRT

used to compensate for missing tissue and variation in the breast separation. Although conventional 3D planning and forward-planned IMRT are both techniques that aim to create a homogeneous dose distribution in the breast by compensating for irregular tissue, the key difference between the two techniques is that with 3D planning, the compensation is decided by a wedge having fixed dimensions, whereas with forward IMRT, it can be customized for each patient throughout the breast, leading to more homogeneous dose distributions with the latter. This customization with forward-planned IMRT can be achieved using multiple static multi-leaf collimator (sMLC) segments to deliver IMRT. Since contouring of the target and critical organs is not required, forward planning IMRT is less time consuming to plan than inverse planning IMRT, making it the popular choice for large-scale implementation in many centers.

As with inverse-planned whole breast IMRT, the field arrangement utilized for forward-planned whole breast IMRT is the same as that for standard 3D conformal planning with two opposed tangential beams. A 3D dose distribution is first calculated for equally weighted open fields (i.e., without any beam modifiers). Since the fields are open, there is no beam modulation, and the dose distribution in the breast as a result is generally inhomogeneous. Isodose surfaces within the breast are projected in the beam's eye view (BEV) of the medial or the lateral field. These isodose surfaces typically range from 100 to 120 %. MLC segments are designed to block these surfaces allowing the customization of tissue compensation, as indicated in Fig. 7.4a, b. Each segment is assigned a weight, and a dose distribution is calculated. Segment weights are optimally adjusted so that hotspots are minimized without compromising adequate coverage to the breast tissue. Lung block segments are also introduced in both the medial and lateral tangential fields to help reduce dose to the ipsilateral lung. A comparison of the dose distributions for a case planned with forward IMRT versus standard wedges is shown in Fig. 7.4c, revealing the dosimetric superiority of the former. The use of forward-planned IMRT results in smaller hotspots compared to using wedges without compromising coverage to the breast tissue.

Comparison of the dose distribution of inverse-planned tangential field IMRT versus forward-planned IMRT/field in field with tangents is shown in Fig. 7.4d. As shown in the comparison of DVHs in Fig. 7.4e, f, both planning techniques show no difference in PTV coverage and dose homogeneity throughout the breast nor in the sparing of the underlying ipsilateral lung. Unlike inverse-planned IMRT, which can require up to approximately 100 MLC segments per beam to deliver radiation, forward planning IMRT requires a total of only 6–8 MLC segments. Most of the dose is delivered using the open field. With inverse planning IMRT, the monitor units (MU) are known to increase by a factor of 2–3 compared to 3D. Higher MU are a concern for a rise in total body exposure due to leakage radiation and thereby potentially increase the risk for secondary cancers. With forward-planned IMRT, however, the MU are much lower than with inverse planning due to reduced MLC segments needed to deliver the radiation and are comparable to those obtained with standard wedge planning. This is another reason why forward-planned IMRT is preferred over both inverse-planned IMRT as well as 3D conformal techniques for whole breast radiation.

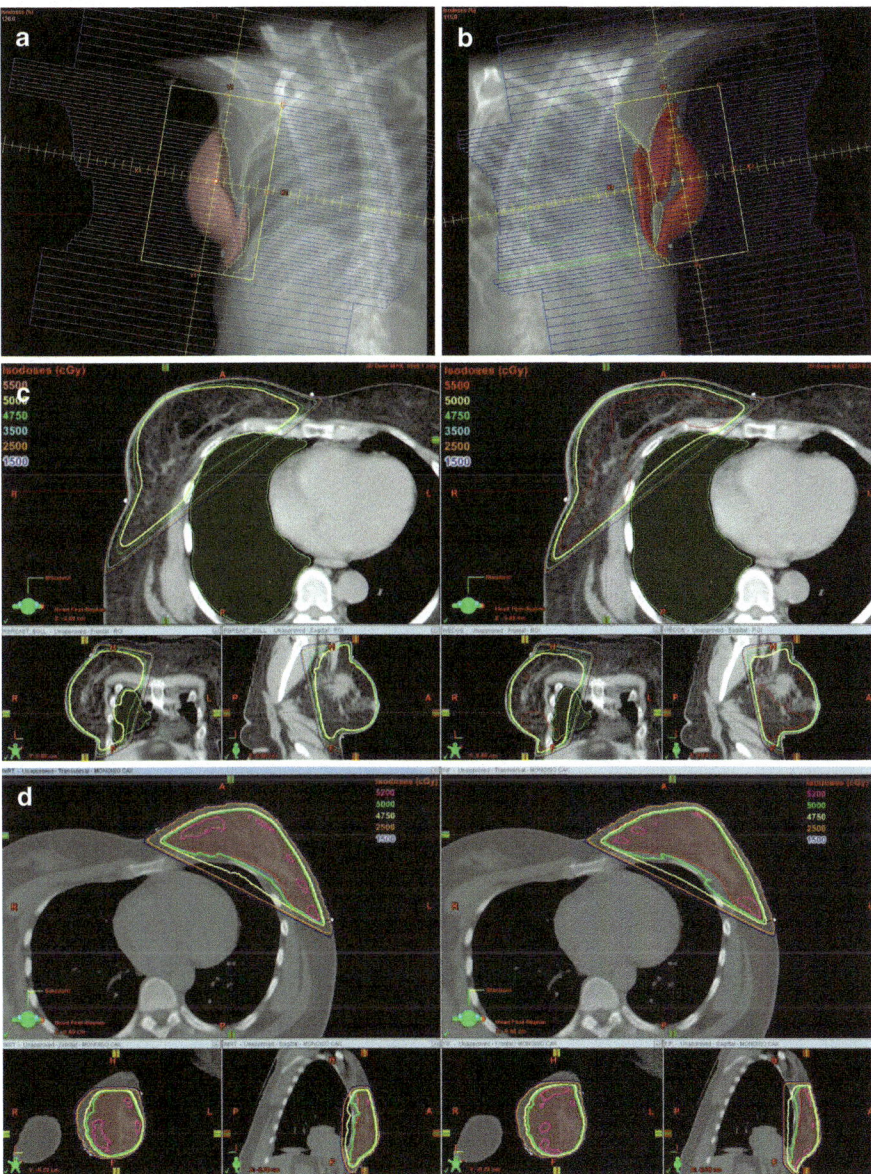

Fig. 7.4 (**a**) Beam's eye view of MLC segment that blocks the 120 % open-field isodose surface. (**b**) Beam's eye view of MLC segment that blocks the 115 % open-field isodose surface along with a lung block segment. (**c**) Comparison of dose distributions in the axial, coronal, and the sagittal planes for a forward-planned IMRT on the left versus the same case planned using standard wedges on the right. (**d**) Comparison of dose distributions in the axial, coronal, and the sagittal planes for tangential inverse-planned IMRT on the left versus tangential forward-planned IMRT/field in field on the right. (**e**) Dose-volume histogram (DVH) comparing PTV coverage for the case planned in (**d**) with field-in-field/forward-planned IMRT versus inverse-planned IMRT. (**f**) Dose-volume histogram (DVH) comparing dose to the ipsilateral lung for the case planned in (**d**) with field-in-field/forward-planned IMRT versus inverse-planned IMRT

Fig. 7.4 (continued)

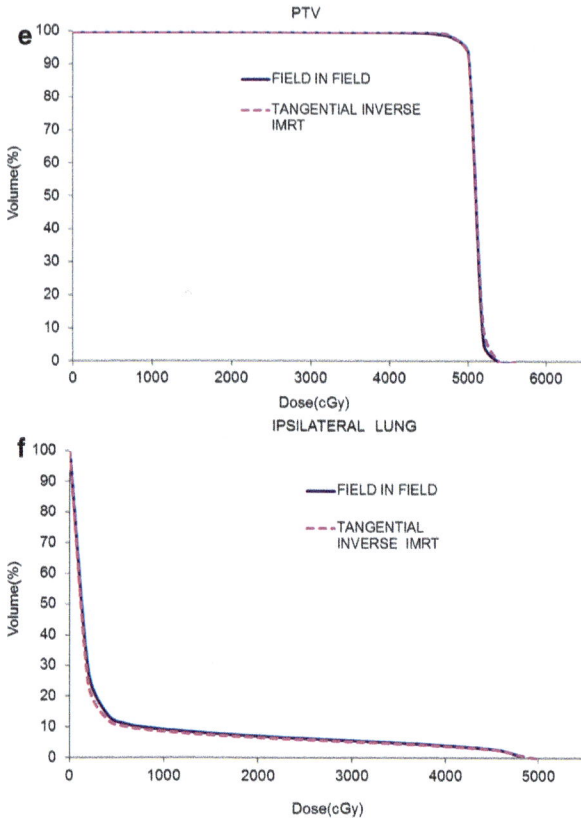

7.3   Simplified IMRT

Simplified IMRT, or sIMRT, is another form of IMRT that was developed at MSKCC in order to treat the whole breast [16, 17]. By using standard tangential fields in order to define the treatment volume, this method of IMRT also does not require contouring, which facilitates the planning process for implementation at a high-volume center. The optimization focuses purely on delivering a uniform dose to the breast. Each tangential beam is modeled as combination of multiple small beamlets or "pencil beams." In this method, the midpoints of the breast are determined from line segments parallel to the posterior edge of the tangential fields that intersect the treatment volume. Every pencil beam in a given tangent delivers 50% of the prescription dose to the midpoint, with the remaining 50% of the dose at this point being delivered by the corresponding pencil beam from the opposing tangential field as shown in Fig. 7.5. This technique mimics an electronic tissue compensator. However it is unique to the MSKCC's homegrown treatment planning system, therefore limiting widespread implementation.

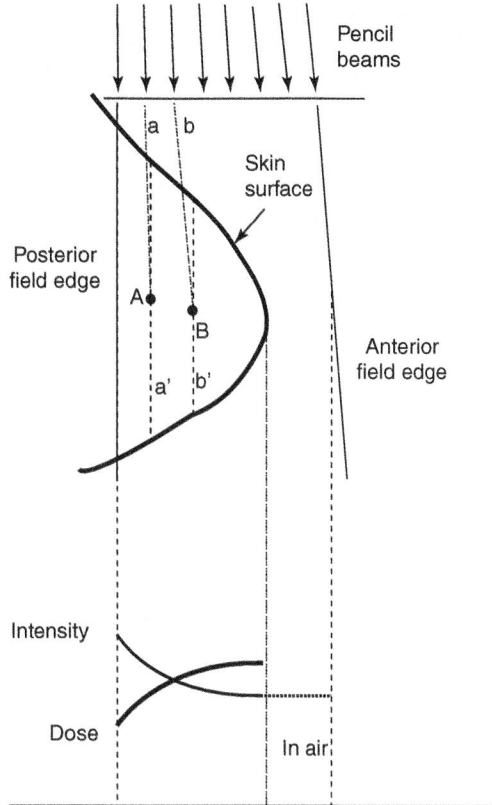

Fig. 7.5 The pencil-beam algorithm used in simplified IMRT technique for whole breast radiation at MSKCC

7.4   Multibeam IMRT for the Breast/Chest Wall and Comprehensive Nodal Irradiation

Treatment planning for comprehensive nodal radiation is more complex than whole breast radiation because it consists of treating the breast and/or chest wall along with regional nodes which include the supraclavicular, infraclavicular, axillary levels I and II, and internal mammary nodes (IMNs). Compared to patients with early-stage breast cancer who may be treated to the whole breast alone, patients with more advanced breast cancers typically require coverage of the chest wall, axillary, and supraclavicular lymph nodes and in some cases, the IMNs. Several conventional techniques using 3D conformal planning have been investigated for regional nodal irradiation (RNI) and are described in Chap. 3 [18]. Depending on the anatomy of the patient and goals for target tissue coverage, the treatment technique must be individualized in order to achieve the most optimal breast/chest wall and regional nodal coverage, while minimizing lung and heart exposure.

Over the past decade, the increased use of contralateral prophylactic mastectomies and bilateral breast reconstruction has also complicated the treatment planning of patients requiring RNI [20]. Ohri et al. [21] have shown that patients who receive

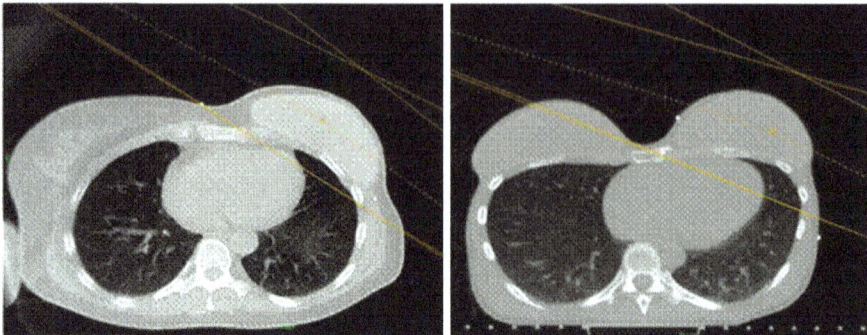

Fig. 7.6 Challenges of treatment delivery with tangential beams are demonstrated in patients with unilateral (*left*) and bilateral (*right*) implants

Fig. 7.7 A CT slice indicating a typical 3D conformal beam arrangement for a left-sided implant reconstruction case where the coverage of the implant and the IMNs requires a significant inclusion of the heart and the ipsilateral lung

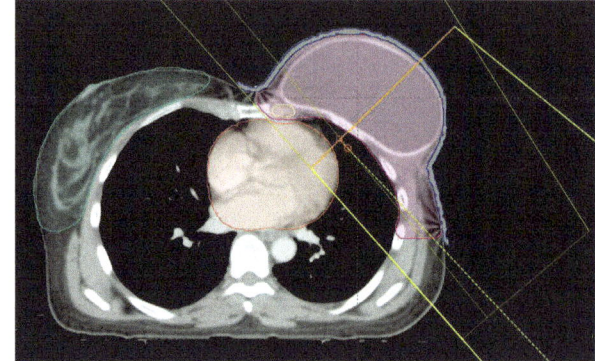

breast reconstruction and require radiation to the IMNs have a significantly increased heart and lung dose than those without reconstruction and requiring the same treatment. In patients with bilateral breast implants, the proximity and hence the potential exposure of the contralateral side to the radiation treatment fields are often unavoidable (Fig. 7.6). Ho et al. [22] demonstrated that in patients with bilateral implants, radiation to the IMNs was an independent predictor for increased dose to the heart, the lung, and the contralateral implant. Figure 7.7 shows an example of a case where adequate coverage of the chest wall and the IMNs with tangential beams/ partially wide tangents may result in significant inclusion of the heart and/or the ipsilateral lung. The mean heart dose (MHD) for this case was noted to be 14 Gy, while the ipsilateral lung V20 Gy was 45 % with 3D conformal planning. Both these dosimetric values are higher than those acceptable for a clinically viable plan. Multibeam IMRT was developed to resolve this treatment dilemma [7, 19]. Multibeam IMRT employs 9–11 beams equally spaced through a 190–220° sector angle around the target volume, which includes the breast/chest wall and regional nodes, as indicated in Fig. 7.8. Details on contouring and outlining of the PTV can be referred to in Chap. 4. Typically 3–5 mm bolus is placed on the breast/

Fig. 7.8 CT slice indicating 11-field IMRT technique with the orientation of 11 beams equally spaced within a sector angle range of 190–220° around the treated reconstruction with IMNs

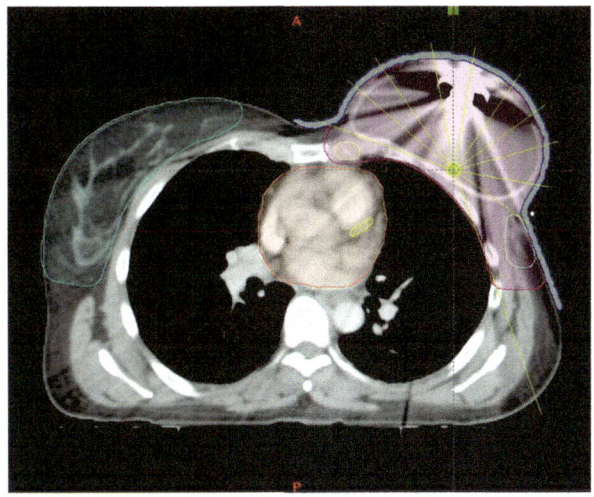

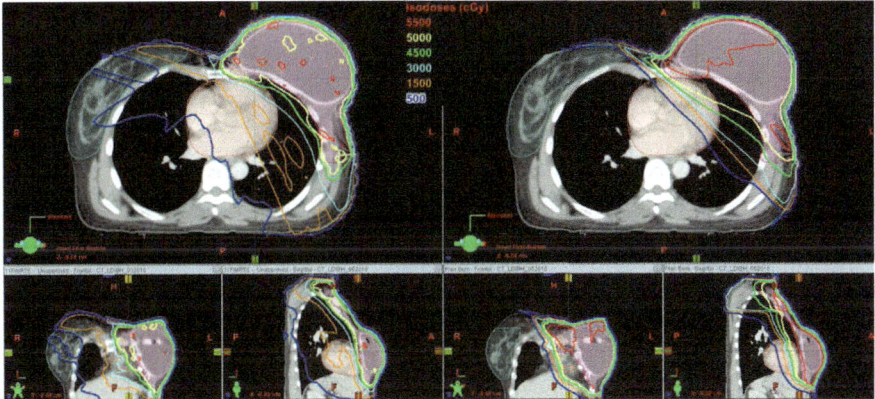

Fig. 7.9 Dose distribution of an 11-field IMRT plan compared to a partially wide tangent technique used to treat the breast/chest wall and IMNs

reconstructed chest wall to improve coverage to the surface of the chest wall or skin. This bolus is attached to the treatment fields and is taken into consideration during plan optimization and dose calculation. The advantage of using multiple beams in a "fan shape" around the target is its ability to produce conformal coverage to the target while carving out the high doses around critical organs, namely, the heart and the lung. A significant reduction in volumes of the heart and the ipsilateral lung receiving 30 Gy or more has been shown compared to standard 3D conformal techniques [7]. In Fig. 7.9 is a comparison of the dose distribution for the reconstructed chest wall case of Fig. 7.7 requiring RNI using 11-field IMRT versus conventional planning (partially wide tangents used in this case). With multibeam IMRT, the MHD was reduced to 8 Gy compared to 14 Gy with the 3D conformal plan, while the ipsilateral lung V20 Gy was reduced to 33 % compared to 45 % with the 3D conformal plan. Moreover with breath-hold techniques, the dosimetric sparing of both the heart as well as the lung can further be improved as will be discussed in the later sections in this chapter.

Despite the numerous dosimetric advantages of multibeam IMRT, an important caveat with this technique is also the increase in low dose that is delivered to the thorax. As shown in Fig. 7.9, although the higher isodose levels ($\geq$30 Gy) to the heart and lung are more limited with multibeam IMRT than with 3-D conformal planning, there is an increase in the volume of normal tissues encompassed by lower doses such as 15 and 5 Gy. This phenomenon of "low-dose bath" to the chest is unavoidable with IMRT, given the entry and exit of the multiple beam arrangements. In a clinical trial of locally advanced breast cancer patients treated with multibeam IMRT at MSKCC, only 3% of patients developed clinically detectable pneumonitis when the V20 Gy of the ipsilateral lung was limited to $\leq$30% [23]. All patients on this trial had a lung V05 Gy of 100%. Although there is little data to support the concern that this low dose may increase the risk of developing radiation-induced secondary malignancies in breast cancer survivors, it is not an unreasonable concern. Therefore, multibeam IMRT should only be utilized in high-risk breast cancer patients who require comprehensive nodal irradiation but cannot achieve an acceptable treatment plan with conventional techniques, either due to the extent of their disease or because of challenging anatomies.

7.4.1 Dose Constraints for Target and Normal Tissue

Dosimetric planning guidelines for multibeam IMRT developed at MSKCC via IRB-approved protocols are shown in Table 7.1. Our constraints were initially developed from a protocol described by Goddu et al. in 2009 [24] and have been refined over the past 7 years. In patients who are receiving prophylactic treatment of the IMNs, the priorities in the optimization are to cover the IMNs such that at least 95% of its volume receives 100% of the prescription dose and the PTV D95 and V95 $\geq$95% without compromising the constraints on the critical organs indicated in the table. Although the D95 for gross IMN disease is $\geq$90% for patients who require prophylactic treatment of the IMNs, the priorities in the optimization may be adjusted so as to cover 100% of the IMN volume with the full prescription dose in cases where there is gross disease in the IMNs that require full coverage.

The mean heart dose (MHD) parameters with multibeam IMRT also differ, depending on the laterality of the tumor and whether or not respiratory gating techniques are utilized. For right-sided tumors, the MHD parameter with multibeam IMRT is not allowed to exceed 5 Gy. For left-sided tumors, the MHD parameter with multibeam IMRT is kept under 9 Gy, but can be further decreased by 1–3 Gy with deep inspiration breath hold (DIBH) [30] (Table 7.1). Notably, heart dose is greatly influenced by coverage of the IMNs and individual patient anatomy and can be reduced to as low as 3–4 Gy with a combination of IMRT and DIBH as will be discussed later. The goal is to include the IMNs while meeting constraints on the MHD, maximum dose, and V25 Gy. Although the risk of ischemic heart disease in patients

Table 7.1   MSKCC dosimetric planning guidelines for breast IMRT/VMAT

PTV D95	≥95 %
IMN D95	≥100 %
PTV D05	≤110 %
Ipsilateral lung V20 Gy	≤33 %; ≤30 % (with DIBH)
Ipsilateral lung V10 Gy	≤68 %; ≤63 % (with DIBH)
Ipsilateral lung mean dose	≤20 Gy; ≤18 Gy (with DIBH)
Contralateral lung V20 Gy	≤8 %
Heart V25 Gy	≤25 %
Heart maximum point dose	≤50 Gy
Heart mean dose, left breast	≤9 Gy (if IMN D95 ≥ 100 %); ≤8 Gy (if IMN D95 ≥ 90 %)[a]
Heart mean dose, right breast	≤5 Gy (if IMN D95 ≥ 100 %); ≤4 Gy (if IMN D95 ≥ 90 %)
Left anterior descending artery maximum point dose	≤50 Gy
Thyroid mean dose	≤20 Gy
Esophagus maximum point dose	≤50 Gy
Brachial plexus maximum point dose	≤55 Gy
Contralateral intact breast mean dose	≤5 Gy
Contralateral implant mean dose	≤8 Gy
Liver (for right sided cases) mean dose	≤10 Gy
Stomach (for left sided cases) mean dose	≤5 Gy; ≤3 Gy (with DIBH)
Cord maximum point dose	≤20 Gy

Assuming a prescription dose of 50 Gy delivered in 25 fractions
[a]Using DIBH, the mean heart dose (MHD) can further be reduced for left-sided cases to within 5–6 Gy, when the IMN D95 ≥ 100 % [30]

treated for left-sided breast cancer has been evaluated by Darby et al. [31] who showed that the risk is proportional to the MHD, it is still not known whether MHD is the best metric. Therefore, even though high doses to the heart can be minimized with IMRT, there could still be side effects from the low dose to the heart generated as a result of increased number of beams, and regardless of what constraints are used, the goal should be to minimize heart dose to the greatest extent possible. While MHD, heart maximum dose, and heart V25 Gy are metrics used at MSKCC, individual institutions have decided upon their own metrics for evaluating the heart dose. Clearly additional research is necessary to determine the optimal metrics.

7.5   Volumetric Modulated Arc Therapy

Volumetric modulated arc therapy (VMAT) is a type of IMRT where the radiation delivery is much faster and requires considerably fewer monitor units (MU), making it a more convenient modality for radiotherapy planning and delivery.

Moreover, with reduced MU, there is also a decrease in total body exposure due to leakage radiation. Unlike static field IMRT, where radiation is delivered from a fixed number of gantry angles, it is delivered continuously over an arc range with VMAT. The intensity of the beam in VMAT is modulated as a function of gantry angle, MLC speed, and the dose rate of the linear accelerator (LINAC). Treatment can be delivered within 1–3 arcs of rotation, with each arc taking under 2 min to deliver. Although the concept of VMAT was first described in 1995 [25], its commercial implementation has only taken place within the past decade. The application of VMAT for locoregional radiotherapy of left-sided breast cancer is relatively new [26]. PTV and OAR contours are the same as in multibeam IMRT. The angle at which the largest separation of the PTV is projected in the beam's eye view (BEV) is chosen. The largest separation often tends to be >15 cm. Due to limitations on the MLC leaf travel within an individual field (which is a maximum of 15 cm on certain linear accelerators), the PTV needs to be covered by a minimum of two fields as shown in Fig. 7.10a. To allow for a smooth transition of dose, the fields overlap at the isocenter by 2 cm. The collimator angle is set to 0°. Each field is an arc whose range is around 190–220° similar to 11-field IMRT as shown in Fig. 7.10b. Both arcs are simultaneously optimized. In the optimizer, the gantry motion is modeled as a number of discrete angular segments and the MLC aperture/shape for each segment is optimally determined for each gantry angle. Variables that are controlled to optimally determine these apertures are the dose rate, the speed of the MLC leaves, as well as the speed of the gantry. VMAT can achieve similar PTV coverage and sparing of organs at risk with a much shorter delivery time and MU compared to IMRT [26]. Figure 7.11 shows a comparison of the dose distribution with 11-field IMRT versus 2-arc VMAT for a left-sided breast cancer patient receiving regional nodal radiation. The monitor units (MU) required for delivery with

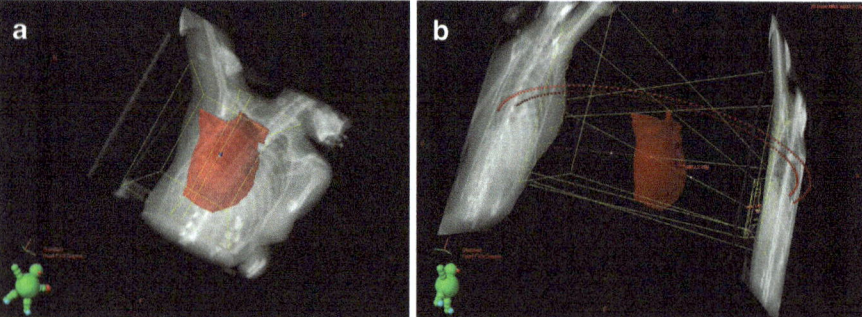

Fig. 7.10 (a) Beam's eye view of the two treatment fields with a 2-cm overlap. These two fields together cover the volume-rendered PTV that combines the breast/chest wall along with all the regional nodes. (b) Two partial VMAT arcs of sector angle range 190–220°. One arc rotates clockwise and the second arc rotates counterclockwise

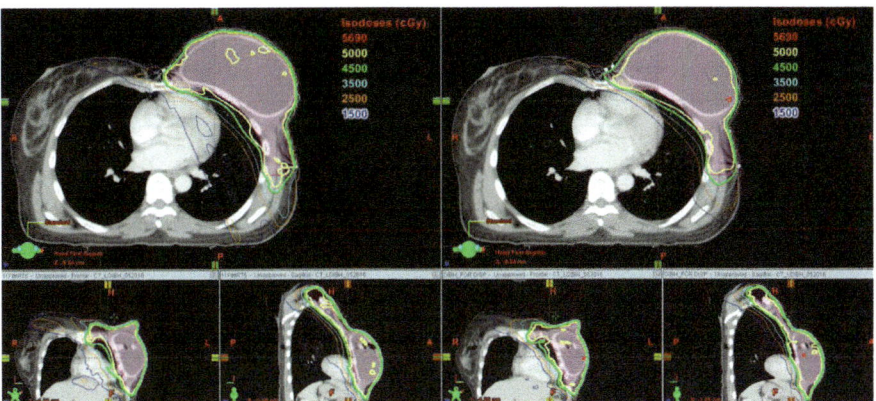

Fig. 7.11 Comparison of the dose distribution with 11-field IMRT in the axial, coronal, and sagittal planes on the left side versus 2-arc VMAT for the same case requiring regional nodal radiation

VMAT are approximately one-third of that required for IMRT. The reduced MU and number of treatment fields contribute toward a faster treatment delivery with VMAT, which enables the utilization of this modality with respiratory gating techniques.

There are additional considerations when choosing between IMRT and VMAT. In cases where RNI is performed, it is necessary to accommodate for variation in treatment due to setup uncertainty and patient breathing and for swelling of breast tissue during treatment. In IMRT planning, the uncertainties introduced by these variations can be overcome by extending the optimal fluence outside the body contour after optimization is completed. Certain treatment planning systems offer a tool referred to as the "skin flash" tool that allows this extension to accommodate for these uncertainties. VMAT planning, however, does not allow the accommodation for skin flash to account for any of these uncertainties. Although the use of artificial bolus in the optimization process would in theory allow for movement of the breast/chest wall during treatment and has been discussed [26], the actual implementation of this technique has not yet been validated. Given the inability of VMAT to accommodate for skin flash, VMAT use is limited to unreconstructed patients or patients with implants or tissue expanders at MSKCC, under the assumption that the degree of swelling would be minimal in patients with breast prostheses or absence of reconstructions, compared to patients with intact breast tissue.

The position of the ipsilateral arm of the patient during treatment can show considerable variation between fractions, as illustrated in Fig. 7.12. Because this can significantly impact the accuracy of dose delivery [27], arm avoidance (AA) VMAT planning technique has been developed at MSKCC [28]. Figure 7.13 shows the details of the field arrangement with AA VMAT.

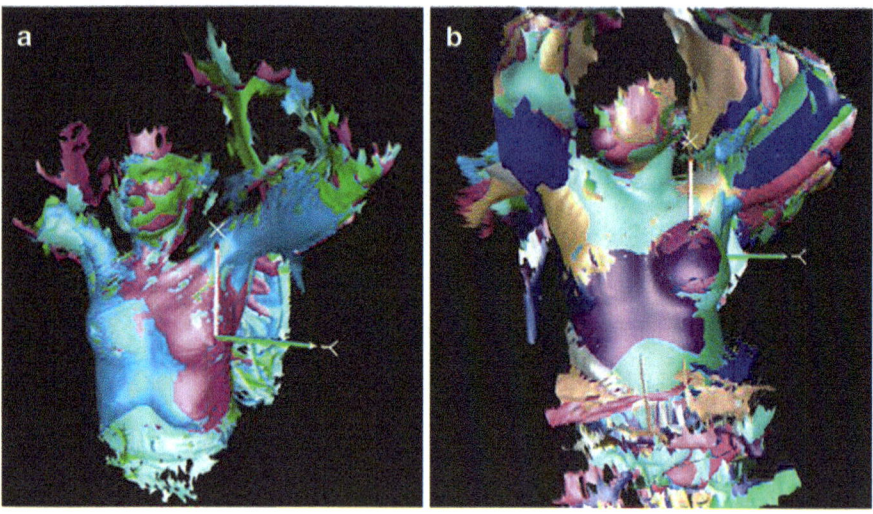

Fig. 7.12 Treatment arm position variation between patients and treatment sections. (**a**) Overlay of 5 surface models which have smaller variation. (**b**) Overlay of 15 surface models which have larger variation. Both patients were immobilized in a Civco® breast board

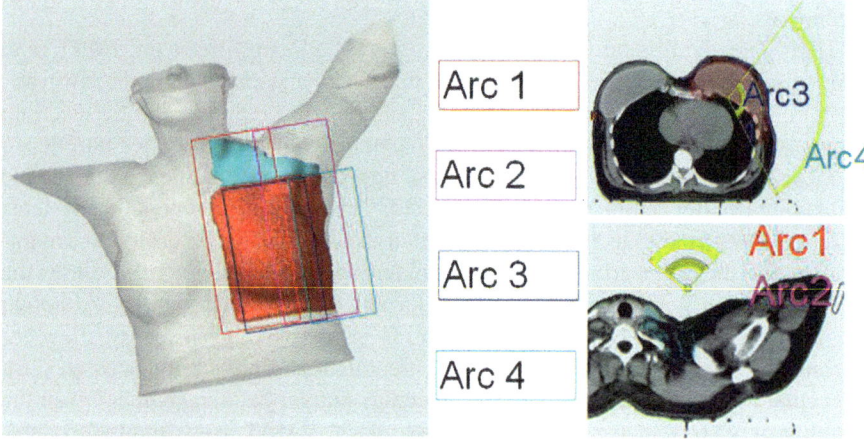

Fig. 7.13 Example of arc geometry for arm avoidance VMAT planning. Two long arcs (Arc1 and Arc2) mainly in the anterior direction and avoiding entering the ipsilateral arm cover the supracla-vicular part and medial chest wall part of the PTV. Two shorter arcs (Arc3 and Arc4) inferior of the ipsilateral arm and extending posteriorly cover the chest wall part of the PTV

7.6   Deep Inspiration Breath Hold (DIBH) with VMAT

Compared to conventional planning for RNI, both VMAT and IMRT have demon-strated the advantage in reducing volume of the heart covered by high doses, namely, the V20 Gy and V40 Gy [7, 26]. However, both these techniques still expose a higher volume of surrounding normal tissue to low dose levels, such as V05 Gy. In addition, the MHD is a parameter of heart dose that clinicians and dosimetrists both strive to minimize to the lowest value possible. Deep inspiration breath hold (DIBH) is a technique that has been applied to maximize the distance between the chest wall and heart allowing for adequate treatment of the breast and underlying chest wall while minimizing irradiated cardiac volume (see Chap. 6) [29]. Combining IMRT with DIBH can therefore potentially provide a cumulative benefit in reduction of MHD and V05 of the lungs for this group of patients. The implementation of breath-hold techniques with multibeam IMRT is impractical, since it would considerably prolong the treatment delivery if a patient were to hold her breath with every field. VMAT, however, due to its shortened delivery time, enables the integration of breath-hold techniques. At MSKCC, DIBH has been utilized in breast cancer patients receiving left-sided comprehensive RNI with VMAT. In a study of 10 patients receiving left-sided RNI, a combination of VMAT and DIBH reduced MHD on average by 3 Gy but also helped to reduce the volumes of the heart and lung covered with 5 Gy isodose line by as much as 30 %, compared to free-breathing DIBH plans performed on the same patients [30]. Hence, the use of DIBH is strongly recommended as an adjunct modality to VMAT when treating left-sided breast cancer patients requiring RNI.

7.7   Simulation

The radiotherapy treatment planning process starts at the time of simulation, where the patient position is set to the anticipated position for treatment planning. The rule of thumb for patient positioning includes (1) easy access by radiation beams without passing through unnecessary normal tissue or causing collision with the gantry, couch, or patient, (2) a comfortable position with an immobilization device that enables the patient to lie still in supine position during treatment, and (3) a reproducible approach with body tattoos, body-couch index, and image guidance to facilitate patient setup at treatments. A three-dimensional (3D) computed tomography (CT) image of a patient at the treatment position will be acquired, which is essential for IMRT planning. Additional imaging modalities may be prescribed and acquired to enhance the visualization of a tumor and surrounding normal tissues and to facilitate tumor delineation and localization, including positron emission tomography (PET)/CT, magnetic resonance imaging (MRI), or respiratory-correlated 4DCT images.

Simulation for breast IMRT treatment requires that the patient lies in supine position on a breast board or a body mold, with the torso tilted upward with 5–10° and both arms up. Unlike simulations for conventional 3DCRT where the head can be tilted contralaterally away from the treatment side, the head position is straight for IMRT simulations to ensure reproducibility. A clinician places wire markers around the breast or implant and on the surgical scar. Intravenous contrast may be used at the discretion of the MD in order to better visualize the nodal regions and/or coronary vasculature. Patient alignment is checked with scout radiograph images, followed by CT scanning with a field of view from the chin to about 5 cm inferior to the marked breast tissue. It is essential to ensure that the entirety of both lungs is included in the simulation scan, so that a lung DVH may be subsequently constructed at the treatment planning stage. Free-breathing CT scans of the patient are obtained. The treatment isocenter is placed at the center of the region that is scanned, generally in the region of the lung. In addition, a second isocenter is marked at the level of a typical match line, in case the MD was to decide to use 3D conventional treatment methods instead of IMRT following simulation. Further details on patient alignment and marking have been covered elsewhere.

7.8   Setup Verification

In image-guided radiotherapy (IGRT), patient setup can be verified daily with either 3D surface tracking such as AlignRT or 2D kilovoltage (2DkV) imaging. With AlignRT, the planner prepares setup reference images using the external contour from simulation CT images for surface alignment. With 2DkV imaging, two orthogonal digitally reconstructed radiograph (DRR) images are generated that provide information on alignment of bony anatomy.

Conclusion

The technique of IMRT has been refined over the past 15 years for both early-stage and locally advanced breast cancer. Methods of IMRT delivery and planning vary widely for breast cancer. Whereas forward-planned tangential IMRT is a convenient and favored approach when the whole breast alone is treated, inverse-planned IMRT with multiple beams is required for cases of comprehensive nodal irradiation. Multibeam IMRT permits excellent coverage of the target tissues while limiting high doses delivered to the lungs and heart. However, multibeam IMRT results in larger regions of normal tissue receiving low dose. VMAT is a type of IMRT that has the added advantage of quick treatment delivery, thereby facilitating the ability to integrate respiratory gating methods. These combined treatments have the potential to further reduce the mean heart dose and decrease the region of low dose delivered by IMRT.

References

1. Clarke M, Collins R, Darby S et al (2005) Effects of radiotherapy and of differences in the extent of surgery for early breast cancer on local recurrence and 15-year survival: an overview of the randomised trials. Lancet 366(9503):2087–2106
2. White J, Joiner MC (2006) Toxicity from radiation in breast cancer. Cancer Treat Res 128:65–109
3. Solin LJ, Chu JC, Sontag MR et al (1991) Three-dimensional photon treatment planning of the intact breast. Int J Radiat Oncol Biol Phys 21:193–203

4. Buchholz TA, Gurgoze E, Bice WS, Prestridge BR (1997) Dosimetric analysis of intact breast irradiation in off-axis planes. Int J Radiat Oncol Biol Phys 39:261–267
5. Ahunbay EE, Chen GP, Thatcher S et al (2007) Direct aperture optimization-based intensity-modulated radiotherapy for whole breast irradiation. Int J Radiat Oncol Biol Phys 67(4):1248–1258
6. Bhatnagar AK, Brandner E, Sonnik D et al (2006) Intensity modulated radiation therapy (IMRT) reduces the dose to the contralateral breast when compared to conventional tangential fields for primary breast irradiation. Breast Cancer Res Treat 96(1):41–46
7. Beckham WA, Popescu CC, Patenaude VV et al (2007) Is multibeam IMRT better than standard treatment for patients with left-sided breast cancer? Int J Radiat Oncol Biol Phys 69(3):918–924
8. Cho BC, Schwarz M, Mijnheer BJ et al (2004) Simplified intensity-modulated radiotherapy using pre-defined segments to reduce cardiac complications in left-sided breast cancer. Radiother Oncol 70(3):231–241
9. Pignol JP, Olivotto I, Rakovitch E et al (2008) A multicenter randomized trial of breast intensity-modulated radiation therapy to reduce acute radiation dermatitis. J Clin Oncol 26(13):2085–2092
10. Donovan E, Bleakley N, Denholm E et al (2007) Randomised trial of standard 2D radiotherapy (RT) versus intensity modulated radiotherapy (IMRT) in patients prescribed breast radiotherapy. Radiother Oncol 82(3):254–264
11. Coles CE, Barnett GC, Wilkinson JS et al (2009) A randomised controlled trial of forward-planned intensity modulated radiotherapy (IMRT) for early breast cancer: interim results at 2 years follow-up. Cancer Res 69(24 Suppl):71
12. Evans PM, Donovan EM, Partridge M et al (2000) The delivery of intensity modulated radiotherapy to the breast using multiple static fields. Radiother Oncol 57:79–89
13. Donovan EM, Bleackley NJ, Evans PM et al (2002) Dose-position and dose-volume histogram analysis of standard wedged and intensity modulated treatments in breast radiotherapy. Br J Radiol 75:967–973
14. Hong L, Hunt M, Chui C et al (1999) Intensity-modulated tangential beam irradiation of the intact breast. Int J Radiat Oncol Biol Phys 44(5):1155–1164
15. Kestin LL, Sharpe MB, Frazier RC et al (2000) Intensity modulation to improve dose uniformity with tangential breast radiotherapy: Initial clinical experience. Int J Radiat Oncol Biol Phys 48(5):1559–1568
16. Chui C, Hong L, Hunt M, McCormick B (2002) A simplified intensity modulated radiation therapy for the breast. Med Phys 29(4):522–529
17. Chui C, Hong L, McCormick B (2005) Intensity modulated radiotherapy technique for three-field breast treatment. Int J Radiat Oncol Biol Phys 62(4):1217–1223
18. Pierce LJ, Butler JB, Martel MK et al (2002) Postmastectomy radiotherapy of the chest wall: dosimetric comparison of common techniques. Int J Radiat Oncol Biol Phys 52(5):1220–1230
19. Krueger EA, Fraass BA, McShan DL et al (2003) Potential gains for irradiation of chest wall and regional nodes with intensity modulated radiotherapy. Int J Radiat Oncol Biol Phys 56(4):1023–1037
20. Motwani SB, Strom EA, Schechter NR et al (2006) The impact of immediate breast reconstruction on the technical delivery of postmastectomy radiotherapy. Int J Radiat Oncol Biol Phys 66(1):76–82
21. Ohri N, Cordeiro PG, Keam J et al (2012) Quantifying the impact of immediate reconstruction in postmastectomy radiation: a large, dose-volume histogram-based analysis. Int J Radiat Oncol Biol Phys 84(2):e153–e159
22. Ho AY, Patel N, Ohri N et al (2014) Bilateral implant reconstruction does not affect the quality of postmastectomy radiation therapy. Med Dose 39:18–22

23. Ho AY, Ballangrud AM, Li G et al (2013) Pneumonitis rates following comprehensive nodal irradiation in breast cancer patients: results of a phase 1 feasibility trial of intensity modulated radiation therapy. Int J Radiat Oncol Biol Phys 87(2):S48–S49

24. Goddu SM, Chaudhari S, Mamalui-Hunter M et al (2009) Helical Tomotherapy planning for left-sided breast cancer patients with positive lymph nodes: Comparison to conventional multiport breast technique. Int J Radiat Oncol Biol Phys 73(4):1243–1251

25. Yu CX (1995) Intensity-modulated arc therapy with dynamic multileaf collimation: an alternative to tomotherapy. Phys Med Biol 40:1435–1449

26. Popescu CC, Olivotto IA, Beckham WB et al (2010) Volumetric modulated arc therapy improves dosimetry and reduces treatment time compared to conventional intensity-modulated radiotherapy for locoregional radiotherapy of left-sided breast cancer and internal mammary nodes. Int J Radiat Oncol Biol Phys 76(1):287–295

27. Bert C, Metheany K, Powell SN (2006) Clinical experience with a 3D surface patient setup system for alignment of partial-breast irradiation patients. Int J Radiat Oncol Biol Phys 64(4):1265–1274

28. Kuo L, Ballangrud A, Ho A et al (2015) Comparison of plan quality between arm avoidance (AA) vs non arm avoidance VMAT planning techniques for breast cancer patients with bilateral implant reconstructions receiving postmastectomy radiation. Med Phys 42(6):3380

29. Sixel KE, Aznar MC, Ung YC (2001) Deep inspiration breath hold to reduce irradiated heart volume in breast cancer patients. Int J Radiat Oncol Biol Phys 49(1):199–204

30. Dumane VA, Saksornchai K, Zhou Y, Hong L, Ho AY (2016) "Quantifying the effects of combining deep inspiration breath hold (DIBH) with volumetric modulated arc therapy (VMAT) in breast cancer patients receiving regional nodal irradiation (RNI)", submitted to ASTRO 58th Annual meeting

31. Darby SC, Ewertz M, McGale P et al (2013) Risk of ischemic heart disease in women after radiotherapy for breast cancer. N Engl J Med 368(11):987–998

Techniques for Proton Radiation

8

Nicolas Depauw, Mark Pankuch, Estelle Batin, Hsiao-Ming Lu, Oren Cahlon, and Shannon M. MacDonald

Contents

N. Depauw, PhD
Department of Radiation Oncology, Francis H. Burr Proton Therapy Center, Massachusetts General Hospital, Boston, MA 02114, USA

M. Pankuch, PhD
Medical Physics and Dosimetry, Northwestern Medicine Chicago Proton Center, 4455 Weaver Parkway, Warrenville, IL 60555, USA

E. Batin, PhD • H.-M. Lu, PhD
Department of Radiation Oncology, Francis H Burr Proton Center, Massachusetts General Hospital, Boston, MA, USA

O. Cahlon, MD
Department of Radiation Oncology, Memorial Sloan Kettering Cancer Center, New York, NY, USA

S.M. MacDonald (✉)
Department of Radiation Oncology, Massachusetts General Hospital, Harvard Medical School, Boston, MA, USA
e-mail: SMACDONALD@mgh.harvard.edu

© Springer International Publishing Switzerland 2016
J.R. Bellon et al. (eds.), *Radiation Therapy Techniques and Treatment Planning for Breast Cancer*, Practical Guides in Radiation Oncology,
DOI 10.1007/978-3-319-40392-2_8

8.1   Introduction

In spite of a slow take off within the proton radiation community for breast cancer as a disease site, proton therapy is an increasingly employed radiation treatment alternative to standard photon and photon/electron treatments for both locally advanced and early stage breast cancer [1–3]. Though most patients do well with standard radiation, risks of cardiopulmonary complications and of radiation-induced malignancy are seen in long-term survivors. Breast cancer outcomes compare favorably to most other malignancies. The longevity that these patients are likely to experience leads to a greater concern for late complications. For both patients and physicians, a late chronic side effect attributable to therapy after surviving a cancer diagnosis can be devastating. For breast cancer patients, the most concerning late side effect of radiation is cardiac morbidity and mortality. Cardiac injury from radiation therapy is thought to occur by direct damage to the myocardium and/or to coronary vessels in close proximity to the chest wall. This includes the mid- and distal left anterior descending coronary artery for patients with left-sided breast cancer and right coronary artery for those with right-sided advanced breast cancer receiving radiation to the internal mammary lymph nodes [4, 5]. Darby et al. demonstrated a direct correlation of major cardiac events and mean radiation dose to the heart [6]. Rates of major coronary events increased linearly with mean heart dose (7.4 % per Gray) with no apparent threshold.

The clinical decision to use proton radiation is dependent on several patient- and disease-related factors. The rationale for the use of protons is that the physical properties of protons allow for sparing of tissues beyond the target from being exposed to radiation. This has been demonstrated for several adult and pediatric malignancies. For breast cancer treatment, protons decrease dose to the heart, lung, and soft tissues beyond the target volume. The degree of improvement is dependent on patient anatomy, and though benefit may be seen from avoidance of other soft tissues, the major benefit is predicted to be attributable to cardiac avoidance. Patient factors that may indicate a greater degree of benefit include unfavorable cardiac anatomy, lack of improvement with breath-hold technique, inclusion of the internal mammary lymph nodes, and breast reconstruction that may limit beam angles [7]. Bilateral implants may pose a particular challenge [8]. Figure 8.1 shows a proton plan compared to a photon plan for a patient with locally advanced breast cancer. Protons may also be of benefit for patients that cannot lift their arms into the typical treatment position above their head due to axillary surgery, rotator cuff injury, arthritis, or others. Due to the lack of exit dose, it is not necessary to use a tangent beam arrangement and patients can be treated with their arms down or akimbo.

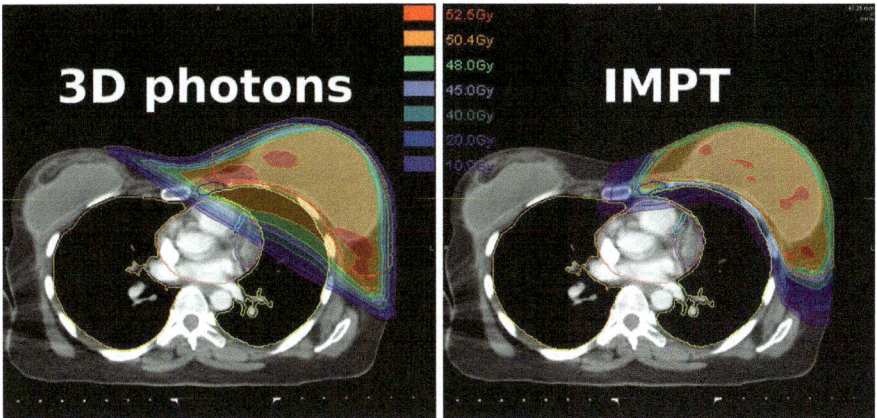

Fig. 8.1 A standard 3D conformal photon plan compared with a proton plan using PBS for a patient with locally advanced breast cancer, bilateral implants, and inclusion of the internal mammary nodes in the treatment field

Despite excellent clinical outcomes reported for the photon experience, target volume coverage as contoured for 3D planning for standard plans is usually less than full with some lymph node targets receiving approximately 60% of full dose and less than 95% coverage with 45 Gy for a dose of 50 Gy [9]. The RTOG created a contouring atlas that has led to an increase in the use of contoured target volumes and avoidance structures for treatment planning available at www.rtog.org/CoreLab/ContouringAtlases/BreastCancerAtlas.aspx. The Radiotherapy Comparative Effectiveness (RADCOMP) randomized trial for proton therapy versus photon therapy for patients with breast cancer receiving radiation to the breast and/or chest wall and regional lymphatics has also created a target and avoidance structure set taking into account special considerations for proton planning available at https://www.rtog.org/CoreLab/ContouringAtlases/RADCOMPBreastAtlas.aspx. Additional benefits from improved dose delivery in anatomically challenging cases and/or sparing of soft tissues may exist.

Proton treatments are prescribed in units of Gray-RBE (RBE=relative biologic effectiveness). This notation designates the higher biologic effectiveness per unit of proton dose. All RBE values are normalized to an expected dose effect when using photons; thus, the RBE for all photon distributions is 1.0 by definition. At the present time for protons, an RBE value of 1.1 is universally and uniformly applied to all proton plans. This value of 1.1 is derived from an average RBE across the entire proton dose range in a large sample of in vivo and in vitro test cell lines [10, 11]. Therefore, for a given prescription dose, the biological effect in the tissue is assumed to be the same for Gy (RBE) of protons as Gy for photons. Further research examining variable RBE is needed and may play a role in future treatment planning in all proton-treated sites.

8.2 Early Stage Breast Cancer

Initial attempts to use protons for breast cancer were focused on accelerated partial breast irradiation (APBI) mainly due to the feasibility based on limited machine time availability. There are many well-accepted forms of PBI delivery including

IORT, interstitial brachytherapy, intracavitary brachytherapy, and external beam radiation (EBRT). Currently, EBRT seems to be the most commonly used form of PBI. Patients treated with APBI are typically patients with early stage breast cancer where recurrence risk is low and serious side effects involving cardiopulmonary tissues are rare. Dosimetric studies have shown that proton therapy reduces the dose of the nontarget breast tissue, heart, and lung. However, given the very low lung and heart doses associated with other forms of PBI, it is unlikely that this advantage would translate into a clinically meaningful benefit. Reports from the University of Michigan and RAPID trial have shown that suboptimal cosmesis is correlated to the exposure to the nontarget breast tissue [12, 13]. Thus, proton therapy can potentially serve as a noninvasive form of PBI with minimal exposure to the nontarget breast tissue, heart, and lung, similar to brachytherapy techniques but without the invasive component and with better homogeneity.

Among the first of the clinical studies was a phase I/II multi-institutional trial of 3D conformal proton PBI in Boston. This initial prescription dose used was 32 Gy (RBE) in twice daily fractions of 4 Gy (RBE), administered over 4 days [14]. Proton APBI did produce significant acute skin toxicity with moderate to severe skin changes in 79 % of patients, and long-term outcomes showed proton APBI appeared to result in higher rates of telangiectasia and pigmentation change [2]. This was attributed to the use of a single field and/or delivery of a single field per treatment used for some patients as patients treated with multiple fields have less skin toxicity. Proton delivery with 3D conformal aperture-/compensator-based delivery can result in full dose to the skin. Based on this experience, a standard of practice to use at least two fields for 3D conformal proton delivery has been adopted. A similar study performed at Loma Linda University using proton APBI sought to administer 40 Gy (RBE) in ten daily fractions of 4 Gy (RBE) [15]. For this trial, two to four fields were used and the 90 % isodose line was maintained within the surface of the skin [16, 17]. Cosmetic results were excellent and the 90 % isodose at the surface of the skin is a reasonable goal to use when planning APBI with scattered protons. Investigators at MD Anderson evaluated multiple proton beam configurations for APBI demonstrating that en face fields provided improved sparing of the breast tissue but a higher skin dose, while tangent fields included more breast tissue and provided better skin sparing, but resulted in a greater amount of setup uncertainty [18].

APBI at most proton centers is done in the supine position with standard breast immobilization techniques, although the group at Loma Linda has had excellent results using a prone setup that has been well described in their publications [15]. The contouring of the tumor bed and CTV should be similar to photon-based EBRT PBI techniques. A PTV margin for setup error needs to be added based on confidence of reproducibility and image guidance capabilities. Beam-specific PTVs to account for range uncertainty are needed for all proton planning. There are no end of range RBE issues that we feel need to be considered for breast PBI. Daily kV imaging to the chest wall and clips is used routinely, and centers with surface mapping capabilities use this to further ensure accurate setup. Several prospective phase II trials are actively recruiting patients including at the University of Pennsylvania and MD Anderson, and there is a multi-intuitional trial through the Proton

Collaborative Group. Long-term follow-up from these trials will better characterize the clinical outcomes of proton PBI using modern techniques.

Protons may also be used for whole breast treatment for early stage disease. A publication from the Paul Scherrer Institute (PSI) in 2009 showed that there is typically little benefit for patients receiving whole breast radiation alone for early stage disease, not requiring any nodal irradiation [19]. Studies and clinical experience have shown that proton therapy has its greatest potential in patients requiring IMN irradiation. However, there are unique cases with unfavorable anatomy where protons can offer a significant dosimetric advantage when treating the breast alone. Several examples of unfavorable anatomy where protons can be beneficial are described below.

In patients with a barrel-shaped chest, standard tangents to cover the whole breast can lead to significant lung exposure. There are cases where the ipsilateral V20 for tangent beams to treat the breast can be as high as 20–25 %. Because the inability to sculpt the high-dose isodose lines, the V30 and V40 in these cases are also close to 20 %. Proton therapy can reduce the lung doses by 50–90 % (Fig. 8.2). The clinical significance of this type of reduction needs to be better studied, but if minimizing lung dose is a priority, protons can significantly do so in some cases.

There are patients in whom the heart hugs the chest wall and avoiding the heart with photons or electrons is very difficult. DIBH can often help but DIBH is still

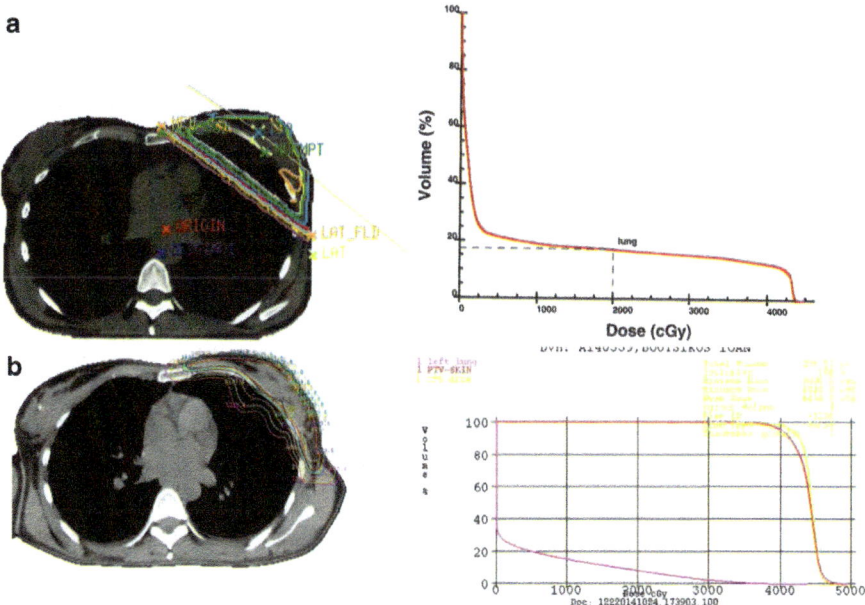

Fig. 8.2 Left whole breast RT with DIBH. Early stage left breast cancer treated with proton therapy for lung sparing. (**a**) Isodose lines and DVH for photon tangents. (**b**) Isodose lines and DVH for uniform scanning proton plan. Comparison of the DVHs shows that the ipsilateral V20 is reduced from 18 to 8 %, V30 from 18 to 2 %, and V40 from 17 to 0 %

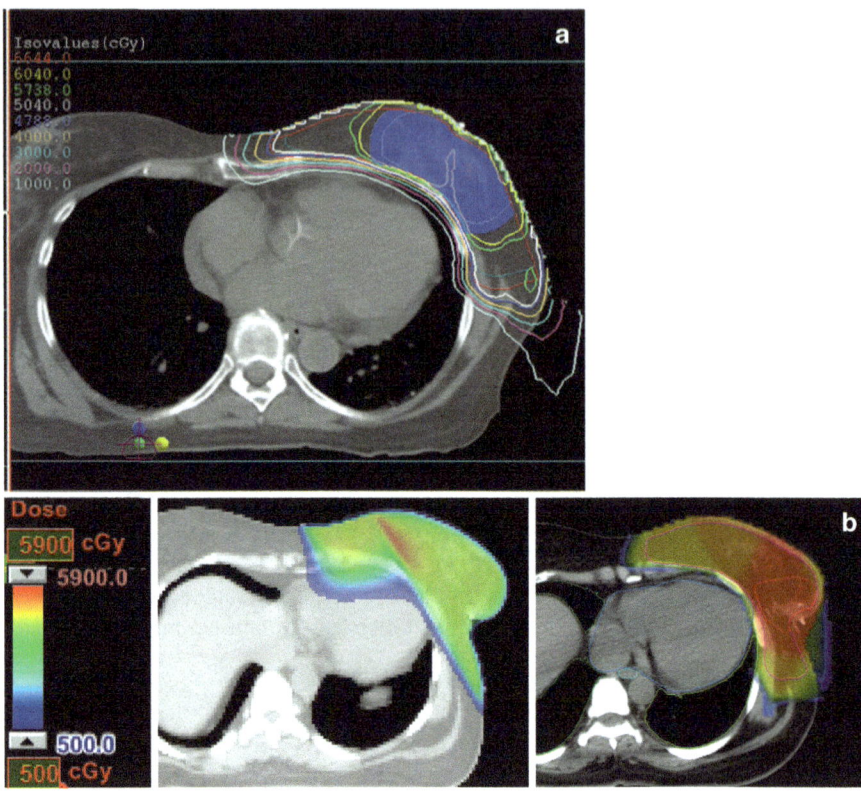

Mean heart dose 3.9 Gy   Mean heart dose 0.2 Gy

Fig. 8.3 L breast treatment for patient that did not tolerate DIBH. (**a**) Tangent fields would have resulted in large portions of the LAD and left ventricle receiving high dose (*red line*). Proton therapy achieved good coverage with near-complete cardiac sparing, with a mean heart dose of 0.3 Gy. (**b**) No displacement of the heart with DIBH so tangent fields resulted in significant exposure to LAD and LV. Thus combined electron/photon plan generated with electron field used to treat the medial breast tissue. No IMN coverage. Mean heart dose still 3.9 Gy with this technique. Patient was therefore simulated for proton therapy, and strong target coverage was achieved with near-complete cardiac sparing with mean heart dose of 0.2 Gy

only available at very few radiation facilities across the country. In addition, there are patients in whom DIBH does not displace the heart and that derive no dosimetric advantage with DIBH and some patients who cannot tolerate DIBH. Figure 8.3 shows an example two of such cases.

In cases with tumor beds located in the medial aspect of the breast, a shallow tangent angle is often needed to obtain strong coverage of the medial breast tissue and adequate margin on the tumor bed. In these cases, there is significant dose being delivered to the contralateral breast (Fig. 8.4). In a young patient with a long life expectancy, this could be associated with an increased risk of contralateral breast cancer.

Skin dose is an important consideration and scanning techniques (explained later in this chapter) may allow for skin sparing. The reported outcomes published thus

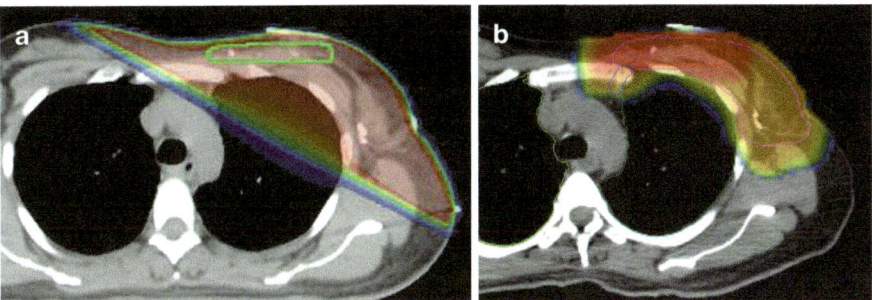

Fig. 8.4 Although the heart was well displaced, because of the location of the tumor bed (*green contour*) in UIQ, there was still significant spillage into the contralateral breast and significant portion of the lung receiving full dose with photon plan (**a**). The proton plan gives excellent coverage of the tumor bed and the IMN chain without increasing dose toe the lung or contralateral dose (**b**)

far from MGH, MSK/Procure, and University of Florida have used passive scattering and uniform scanning (explained later in this chapter) and were associated with reasonable skin toxicity. Longer-term follow-up will be needed to assess for cosmesis, fibrosis, and telangiectasias. A whole breast dose of 45 Gy is frequently favored by the authors, especially if 3D conformal techniques are used, followed by a boost to the tumor bed to a total dose of around 60 Gy. To our knowledge, there are no published reports or large clinical experiences using accelerated fractionation schemes (i.e., Canadian fractionation) for whole breast irradiation with proton therapy, and we have typically used conventional fractionation for these cases.

For patients receiving proton radiation to the breast only, matching fields are typically not required. Depending on the anatomy, a single field can typically encompass the full target volume. For aperture-based/scattered protons, we have typically used two anteriorly obliqued beams for these cases to improve robustness and homogeneity and spread out uncertainties associated with a single beam. With pencil beam scanning techniques, we generally employ a single oblique beam. Technical issues related to treating an intact breast in terms of reproducibility, breast edema, etc., will be reviewed later in the chapter.

8.3   Locally Advanced Breast Cancer

For the treatment of locally advanced breast cancer, it is critical for target and avoidance structures to be accurately contoured. Unlike 3D conformal photon therapy that delivers some dose beyond contoured structures, proton therapy will not deliver dose beyond the contoured structures. For target volume delineation, please refer to the RADCOMP atlas available at https://www.rtog.org/CoreLab/ContouringAtlases/RADCOMPBreastAtlas.aspx. When contouring the chest wall and/or breast CTV, one must take care not to include the ribs as this will lead to an overshooting of dose into the lung. The ribs are not considered to be at risk of harboring microscopic disease. It is therefore appropriate to exclude them as CTV and alternatively use the ribs and the uninvolved intercostal spaces as a stopping region for the proton fields. Lymphatics may be contoured as one volume, but may also be contoured individually as separate levels. The level 1 axilla is often excluded for patients that have undergone an axillary dissection. Though some of the level 2 lymph nodes are also removed in a standard dissection, it is important to realize that the interpectoral nodes (Rotter's nodes) are not typically removed and that more medially located lymph nodes may not be removed. A good guide to what has been dissected is the clips placed in the axilla following a nodal dissection. Figure 8.5 shows contours as delineated by the RADCOMP atlas. The supraclavicular volume can be challenging. It does come in contact with the thyroid gland and esophagus, which should be included as organs at risk (OARs). For proton planning, the RADCOMP atlas extends the supraclavicular volume to meet the internal mammary node volume so that there is a continuous chain rather than a gap between these two volumes. The RADCOMP group also plans for cardiac substructures to be contoured centrally, but substructure guide has been included in the atlas for investigators to use should they wish to delineate these structures (Fig. 8.6).

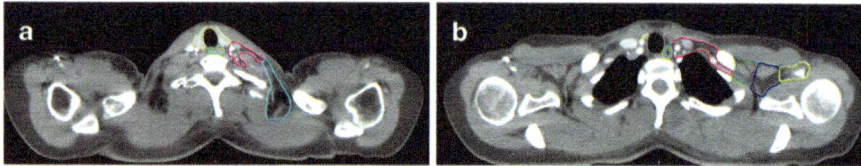

Fig. 8.5 Contours per the RADCOMP atlas (**a**, **b**). The posterior neck (*cyan*) is an optional volume. This is an area that would receive some dose with a standard photon plan but would receive no dose with proton therapy. Some investigators/breast clinicians consider this area potentially at risk for high-risk patients with LABC. The supraclavicular volume is in magenta, level 1 axilla (*yellow*), level 2 axilla (*blue*), and level 3 axilla (*green*). Avoidance structures including the thyroid (*yellow*) and esophagus (*green*) are also shown

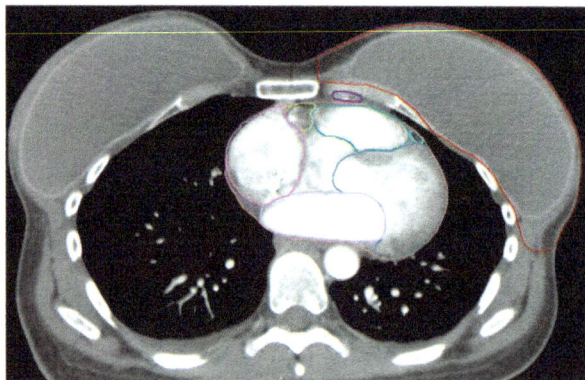

Fig. 8.6 Cardiac contours per the RADCOMP atlas. The LAD shown in cyan and RCA shown in *bright green*. The left ventricle (*denim blue*), right ventricle (*teal*), left atrium (*light purple*), and right atrium (*pink*) also shown. The internal mammary nodes (*dark magenta*) and chest wall (*red*) are also shown in this image

Early results of proton plans for PMRT have been reported with acceptable early toxicity [3, 7]. In addition, several comparative plans using photon techniques compared with 3D conformal passively scattered proton or PBS plans have shown comparable coverage while maximally sparing cardiac and pulmonary structures without sacrificing target coverage. Most studies show superior coverage, improved dose homogeneity, and reduced maximum percentage dose with improved sparing of normal tissues. Delivery techniques are described below.

8.4   Proton Delivery Techniques

The dose deposition of a proton beam is very different than that of photons. High-energy photons deliver their dose with initially a short buildup near the surface than an exponential loss of energy with depth. The depth-dose shape of any high-energy photon field is a result of photon interactions within the media that transfer a portion of the interaction photon's energy to secondary electrons. These energetic secondary electrons then interact within the media and deposit the dose along the secondary electron's path, away from the initial interaction site. Since protons have a charge, they are directly ionizing radiation and a proton depth-dose curve appears very different from those of photons. Protons enter the media and experience a gradual loss of energy along their path. The high mass of the proton (~2000 time greater than that of an electron) allows the proton to move predominantly in the forward direction. As the proton's energy gets lower, the protons begin to transfer its remaining energy at a very high rate until all kinetic energy is transferred to the media. This rapid increase in dose at low energy generates the Bragg peak, characteristic of all heavy particle beams (Fig. 8.7). The higher the incident proton energy is, the deeper the Bragg peak will appear.

The typical linear accelerators used in photon therapy accelerate electrons to kinetic energies ranging from 4 MeV on the low side to a maximum of about 23 MeV. Clinically useable proton kinetic energies vary from ~70 MeV for a Bragg peak edge at 4 cm deep to 250 MeV for a Bragg peak edge at 38 cm deep. The larger mass of the proton, along with the higher energy required to generate a usable clinical beam, is beyond the physical limitations of a current linear accelerator technology, and alternative acceleration systems must be used. There are two types of accelerator systems used for proton therapy: a synchrotron and a cyclotron.

The synchrotron accelerates protons in a fixed ring rotation by boosting the proton's energy in each revolution. The generation of higher-energy protons requires more revolutions to achieve the greater energy. During each rotation the magnets that keep the protons constrained within the ring must be synchronously increased in strength to maintain a stable proton orbit. Once the protons are at the energy needed for treatment, they are "spilled" into the beamline and directed to the treatment room by a series of focusing and bending magnets. Synchrotrons produce beams in a pulsed beam structure requiring a period to "fill" for acceleration and then "spill" into the treatment rooms. A cyclotron accelerates protons within a fixed magnetic field. Low-energy protons are injected into the center of disk-shaped

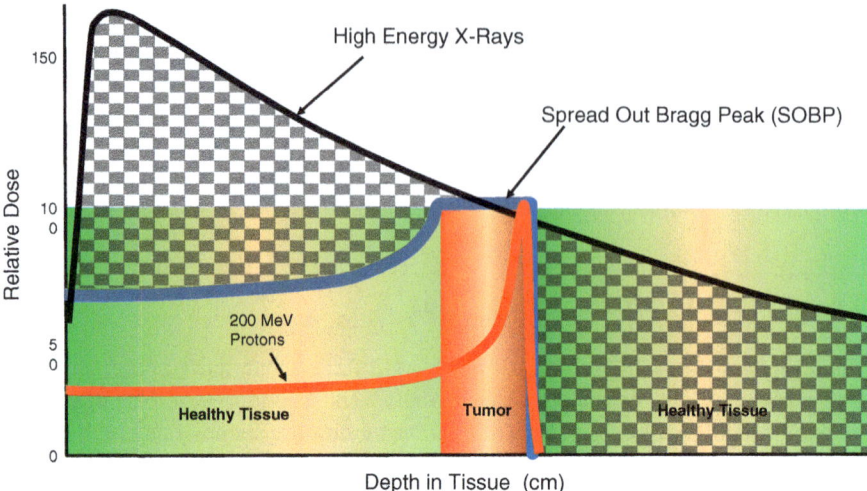

Fig. 8.7 Dose-depth distribution. Photon beam is shown in *green*. Spread-out Bragg peak (SOBP) in *black*. Many individual Bragg peaks combine to form a SOBP. No dose is deposited beyond this region allowing for complete sparing of tissues deep to the target

accelerating cavity and are increased in energy by passing through accelerating cavities place within the disk. The constant magnetic field binds the protons to a circular path within the disk, but in each rotation, the protons gain energy and spiral radially outwards with increasing energy. At the outermost orbit, the protons are "peeled" off and directed down the beamline for clinical use. All protons leaving the cyclotron are at the maximum clinically available energy. Since energies lower than the maximum are most commonly used, the proton beam is directed through a degrader composed of low scattering material that interacts with the protons and lower their energy to the desired clinical energy. The cyclotron delivers a continuous output of protons once the degrader and beamline magnets are set.

Regardless of the accelerator system, the treatment proton beam is directed down an evacuated beamline using a combination of focusing and steering magnets into the treatment nozzle. The function of the nozzle may vary depending on the delivery method used, but in general, the nozzle contains components to spread the beam across the target region, collimate the beam, modulate the beam energy into a spread out Bragg peak (SOBP), and monitor the dose given to the patient. Delivery methods used for breast treatment may include aperture- and compensator-based delivery using SOBP or pencil beam scanning (PBS) delivery.

In SOBP-type treatments, the proton beam from the beamline must be spread in both the lateral direction and the depth direction to cover the entire volume of the target. Spreading of the beam in the lateral direction can be done using double scattering (DS) methods or uniform scanning (US). In DS the beam in the nozzle is passed through two scatterers to passively spread the beam across the target. The use of two scatterers is necessary to maintain proton energy consistency over the entire field. The maximum field size for a passively scattered beam is approximately 25 cm in diameter by projection, but the effective field size with less than 2% of dose heterogeneity is only 22–23 cm. For APBI treatment, such field size limits are not an issue. For irradiation of the intact breast and/or chest wall including regional nodal targets, however, this maximum field size would not be able to cover the entire target volume for most patients. In that case, multiple abutting fields must be used, similar to photon 3D techniques, subsequently mandating the need for daily feathering (e.g., by 1 cm). For breast or chest wall treatments that do not include regional lymphatics, a single field is likely to be sufficient.

An alternative to scattering the beam over the target region is to magnetically wobble the beam in a fixed pattern over the treatment portal to obtain a uniform field. This technique is termed uniform scanning. Uniform scanning generally offers a larger field size limit, up to 30 cm × 40 cm, and can typically cover the entire target volume without the need for field matching. However, without intensity modulation, multiple fields may still be occasionally needed to reduce dose heterogeneity.

The pristine peak of a single Bragg peak is not sufficient to treat most targets in the depth direction, and a combination of Bragg peaks of decreasing energy and decreasing intensity is integrated to generate a dose in depth. This is called the spread-out Bragg peak (SOBP) and is modulated wide enough to cover the entire target area in the depth direction. The spreading of the Bragg peak can be accomplished by running the beam through a stepped modulator wheel which is most commonly used in DS or by layer stacking in US. In either case an increasing amount of modulator material is place in the beam path, degrading the beam energy and pulling back the depth of the Bragg peak. To obtain a uniform dose distribution in depth, the intensity of the shallower peaks needs to be decreased because of the prior contribution of higher-energy peaks. The larger the modulation, or pullback of the SOBP, the larger the skin dose becomes. Modulation width is therefore one of the major factors for controlling skin dose.

SOBP-based delivery using either DS or US makes use of customized portal apertures to collimate the beam to the silhouette of the target (Fig. 8.8). Apertures

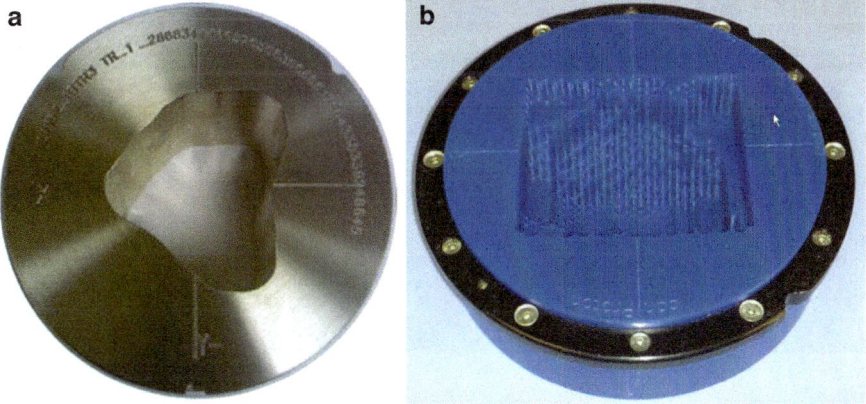

Fig. 8.8 Figures of a patient-specific aperture and compensator. (**a**) Apertures define the field shape in the direction lateral to the beam direction. (**b**) Compensators are used to shape the distal edge to the. Apertures and compensator are unique to every patient and every field

are milled from a high-density material, such as brass, which is thick enough to completely stop all protons outside of the aperture opening. Unlike in linacs, the aperture position is not fixed on most proton systems so the lateral penumbra becomes a variable function of distance to the patient. A large penumbra is preferred when fields are abutted due to field size limitations, but will spread unwanted dose outside of the field where match lines are not present.

Downstream of the apertures, custom compensators are used to further affect the proton energy in order to conform to the distal edge of the target. Compensators are also used to spatially modify the incident proton's energy for tissue inhomogeneities along the anticipated beam path. Although compensators provided distal conformity to the proton beam to allow better sparing of the heart and lung structures, they also can increase skin dose to full prescription in some areas, and toxicities have been observed. Compensators are often made of acrylic or Freemans wax.

Another delivery method, very well suited for breast treatments, is PBS. PBS does not require aperture or compensators to shape the beam, but instead uses scanning magnets to "paint" a distribution of individual spot patterns across the desired treatment field. PBS delivery has full control of spot intensity on a spot-by-spot basis enabling very uniform dose deposition using intensity modulation. PBS fields are delivered one energy at a time, in a method similar to the layer stacking used in US. PBS field can be large, normally 30 cm × 40 cm, except in certain compact systems. As a result, a single PBS field, usually positioned *en face*, is sufficient to cover the entire breast/chest wall and all nodal targets with a homogeneous dose distribution. The power of intensity modulation provided by PBS allows for optimal control of the skin dose over the entire treated area (Fig. 8.9).

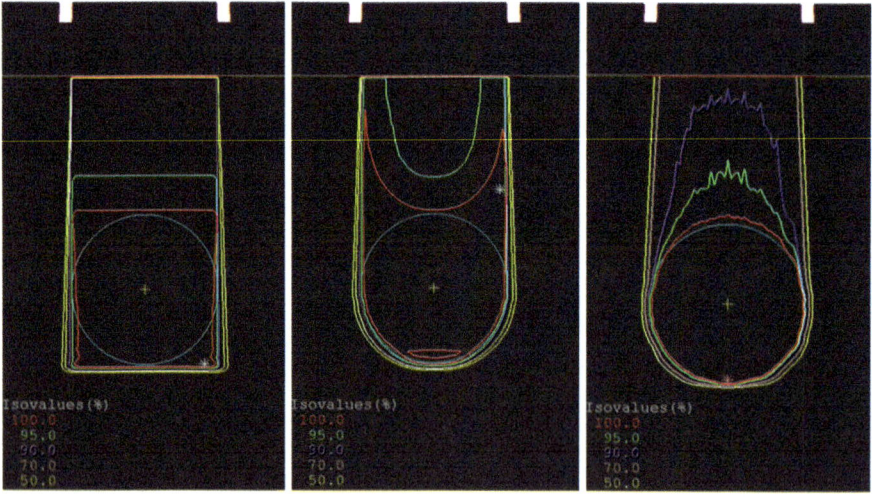

Fig. 8.9 A sphere is treated with a single proton field from the top. (**a**) An uncompensated SOBP. (**b**) A SOBP with a range compensator providing improved distal conformality. Distal dose is displaced from the distal end to the proximal end when using the compensator. (**c**) A PBS beam. PBS allow for distal and proximal shaping of for the added

8.5   Special Considerations

8.5.1   CW Implant

For patients that undergo reconstructive surgery, the breast implant will result in a deeper treatment range and therefore a larger range uncertainty. Measurements should be performed in order to accurately assess the relative proton stopping power ratio (RSP) of the material inside each type of breast implants [14]. A simple measurement consists of irradiating a Bragg peak with known energy/range through a water phantom with and without a fixed amount of the material found in breast implants. The measured range degradation can then be used to more accurately define the RSP of the implant material.

The stoichiometric method is the algorithm most commonly used to obtain RSP from CT simulation Hounsfield units (HU). The inaccuracies in the Hounsfield unit (HU) conversion process for nonhuman-type tissues are an inherent limitation of the stoichiometric method. Directly applying this conversion to the implant material could result in significant errors in RSP values used in planning. For silicone-based implants, for instance, the Hounsfield units found in the breast implants correspond, on average, to RSP of 1.02 based on a clinical conversion curve, as evaluated on ten patients. The range pullback observed through direct measurement of the implant materials, on the other hand, yields a value consistent with a material of 0.92 RSP value, 10 % lower.

During the planning process, the breast implants need to be contoured and their RSP values homogeneously overridden to the measured value. The omission of this correction would result in the treatment planning system computing each pencil beam with a pullback error, translating, in the above example, to a 10 % overshoot during treatment delivery. With the contribution from the breast implants entirely eliminated, the resultant range uncertainties consist only of those found in the real chest wall tissue (minimal thickness) and can therefore be practically ignored.

8.5.2   Plan Robustness

For PBS, beam perturbations arise from multiple sources such as range uncertainties, setup errors, and patient motion (especially breathing motion). As a consequence, the robustness of each field, as well as the overall plan, is an important factor which should be taken into consideration for PBS treatment planning. At the time of redaction, there has not been an exact set of guidelines or methodologies to ensure nor quantify plan robustness. Solutions such as geometrical margins, interpencil smearing, or large hot spots within the target volumes have been suggested but not clinically validated. For now, treatment robustness can only be assessed a posteriori through recomputations of the nominal plan under different scenarios.

This section therefore intends to offer an overview of these uncertainties from a clinical standpoint, looking at DVH deviations from a nominal plan. Nominal plans were based on MGH's PMRT technique as described in Depauw et al. [20].

Additionally, and in order to provide a more useful range of results, these analyses were performed using two specific PBS spot sizes: 8–14 mm (large spot) and 2–5 mm (small spot), respectively, as a function of decreasing energy from 230 to 90 MeV.

8.5.3 Setup Shift Uncertainties

Setup shifts might result in a displacement of the beam along heterogeneities where a large water equivalent path length (WEPL) difference might occur. Such discrepancy could then translate into a significant local under/overshoot of single pencil beams.

The analysis of setup shift uncertainties was performed as a recomputation of nominal plans with the introduction of geometrical perturbations, i.e., shift in patient position. The perturbations were as follow: ± 3 mm along each translation axis (lateral, longitudinal, vertical), ± 2° along each rotation axis (yaw, pitch, roll), and a combination of all aforementioned ± shifts in all six directions simultaneously. DVH data were then generated for each scenario. The composite dose distribution based on the average of the individual shifts was also computed and its DVH generated. Due to the statistical randomness of the setup shifts over the course of a large fractionation scheme, the latter average dose distribution is expected to closely mimic the actual treatment.

The result of this setup shifts uncertainty analysis is presented in Fig. 8.10 as DVH envelopes which correspond to the maximum amplitude from any of the perturbations applied to the nominal plan.

Tumor coverage remains stable in any scenario, hence demonstrating the adequate robustness of the utilized planning approach. Although the effect on most OARs is small, the IMN coverage, as well as the thyroid and esophagus sparing – which are all dosimetrically linked – suffers significantly more from these setup shifts.

As expected, these perturbations have a larger effect on a plan based on a small spot machine when compared to a large spot plan. This is explained by the fact that the amplitude of the shifts is comparable to the size of the beam. The nominal dose distribution with the smaller spot size, however, is far better than the larger spot size plan, and its worst case scenario remains similar to the one of the larger spot size. In both cases, the composite dose distributions based on the average of the individual shifts' doses are remarkably close to the intended treatment. These DVH deviations are therefore considered clinically acceptable, and both plans reasonably robust.

8.5.4 Respiratory Motion Uncertainties

For the breathing motion study, a 4D CT scan of the patient was acquired in addition to the helical planning CT scan performed at quiet/normal respiration. The PBS fields created for the nominal plans were then transferred to each phase of the 4D

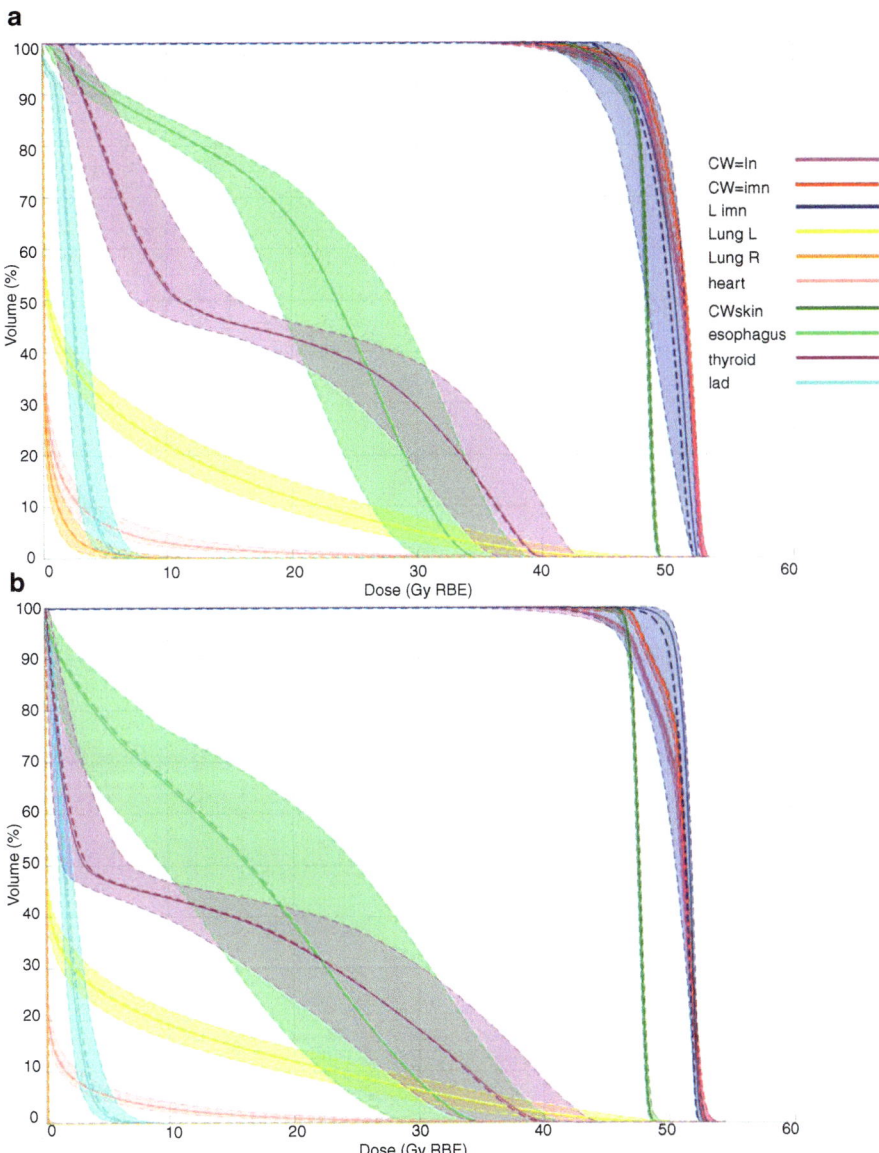

Fig. 8.10 DVH envelopes based on the robustness analysis of the setup shifts (±3 mm, ±2°) performed on a PMRT patient plans (*solid line*): (**a**) 8–14 mm spot (*large*), (**b**) 2–5 mm spot (*small*). The *thick dotted lines* correspond to the composite dose distribution based on the average of the individual shifts' doses

CT scan and the dose distributions recomputed. DVH were generated for each of the ten phases as well as for the total composite dose accumulated through deformable registration, mimicking the actual treatment. Figure 8.11 shows the result of the breathing motion analysis for both the large and small spot plans.

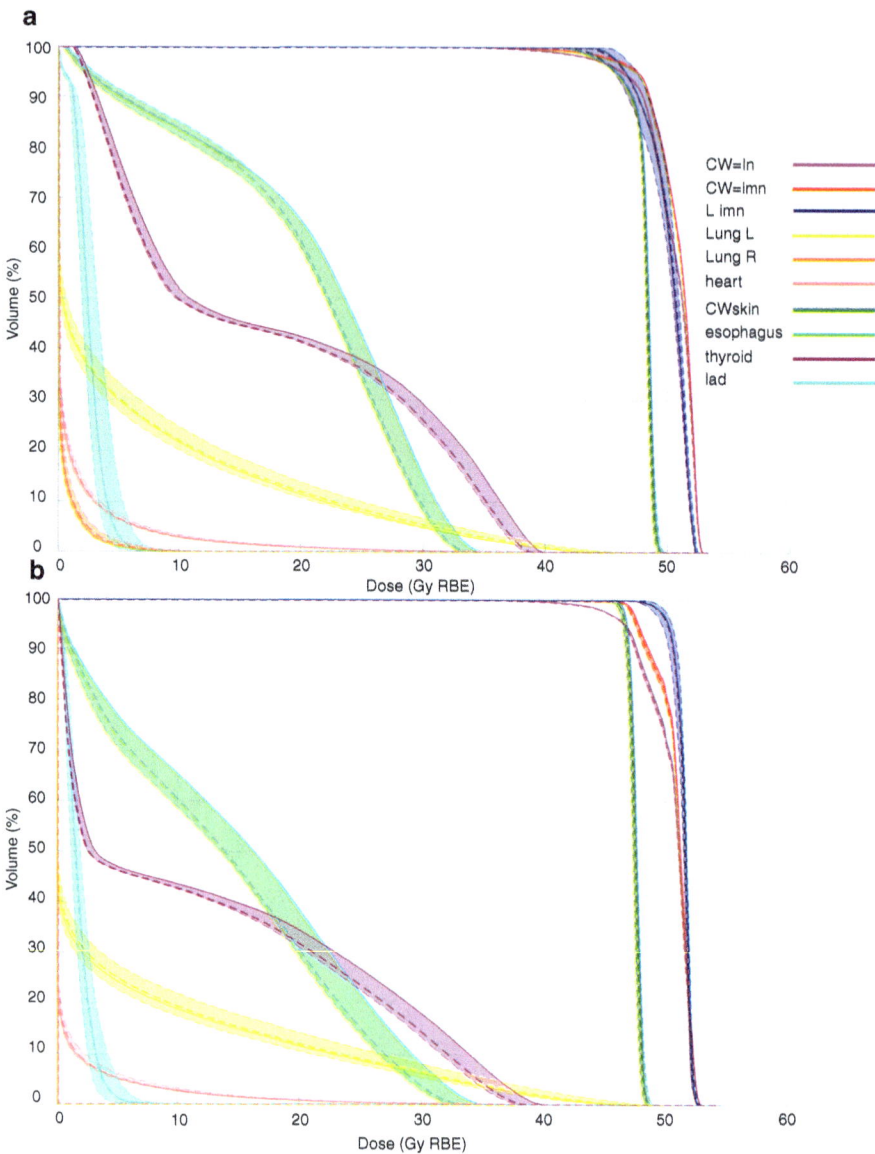

Fig. 8.11 DVH envelopes based on the breathing motion analysis performed on a PMRT patient plans (*solid line*): (**a**) 8–14 mm spot (*large*), (**b**) 2–5 mm spot (*small*). The *thick dotted lines* correspond to the composite dose distribution based on the average of the ten breathing phases' doses

These recomputations resulted in little difference for either machine. These deviations, drastically smaller than the ones observed in the setup shift robustness analysis, are thus believed to be of no clinical concern. Furthermore, the composite dose distributions based on the average of the ten breathing phases' doses – which statistically correspond to the actual treatment – are remarkably similar to the nominal plans.

8.5.5   Range Uncertainties

Range uncertainties represent the main limitation of proton therapy and many research studies aim at improving the issue. These range uncertainties occur due to setup quality, quality of the CT units' conversion to relative stopping powers, beam degradation, etc.

Fortunately, for patients without a breast implant, the chest wall target volumes are very shallow with a required beam range of 3 cm or less. The associated uncertainty is thus only around a millimeter and can be practically ignored, being comparable to uncertainties in CT scanning, contouring, etc.

For patients that undergo reconstructive surgery, however, the implant will result in a deeper treatment range, hence larger range uncertainties. Due to the accurate characterization of the CW implant's material RSP (cf Sect. 8.5.1), the contribution from the breast implants is entirely eliminated. Thus, the resultant range uncertainties consist only of those found in the native chest wall tissue and can therefore be practically ignored.

This point was further highlighted through recomputations of a large spot plan with ±3.5 % range error. The plan consisted of a postmastectomy case without implant entirely treated to 50.4 Gy (RBE). Figure 8.12 gives the resultant DVH bands. Target coverage is very well conserved under either scenario. Naturally, larger discrepancies are observed for the lung and the esophagus which are made of air cavities sitting at the end of range. These effects, however, are not clinically worrisome given the nominal OAR doses. Nevertheless, it is important to note that range uncertainties are systematic, i.e., every single fraction will be delivered with the same error, and therefore must be added to other (random) uncertainties.

8.5.6   Intact Breast Case

Intact breast cases present additional uncertainties over postmastectomy patients with or without implant. Indeed, the range uncertainties are not limited to that of the chest wall (~1 mm) anymore, but to the overall breast tissue thickness. There are also concerns about setup reproducibility and breathing motion. Increased ptosis and/or decreased breast tissue density may be less reproducible, and breathing motion may impact setup to a greater degree with intact breast tissue as compared to an implant (with little motion) or chest wall. Finally, the breast tissue is known to traditionally swell over the course of treatment for conventional photon therapy of intact breast patients.

At the time of redaction, the consensus has been that moderately sized intact breast patients (A/B cups – as appreciated by the physician) or very static (more dense) larger-sized breasts may have less uncertainty for PBS given the aforementioned concerns.

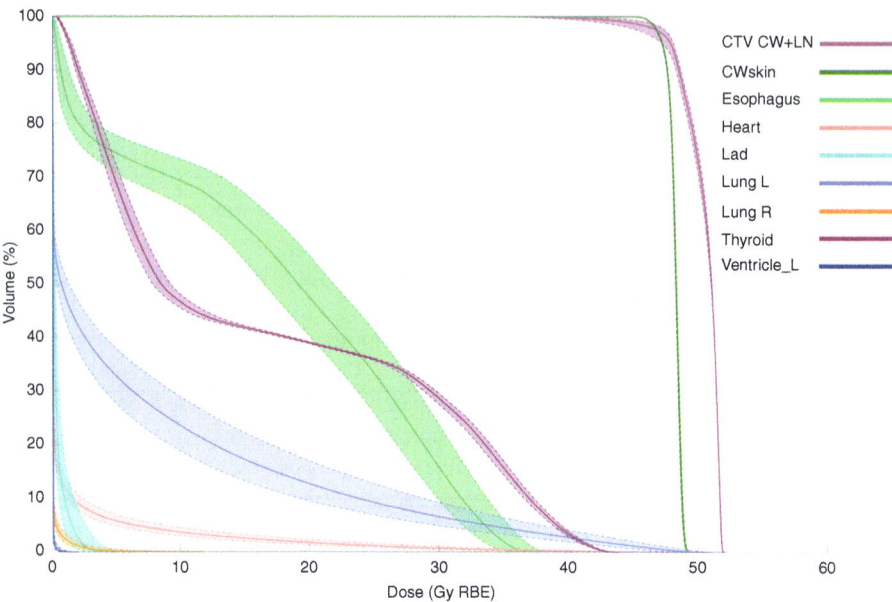

Fig. 8.12 DVH envelopes based on the robustness analysis of range uncertainties (±3.5 %) performed on a PMRT patient's plan without implant (*solid line*)

In order to assess the effect of breast motion a priori, multiple CT simulations were acquired for the first few intact breast patients: one helical CT for planning followed by one 4D CT on the first day and then two additional helical CTs on a second day, with the patient standing up/moving around between scans. The 4D CT set was used to specifically evaluate the pendulum effect as a function of breathing motion, while the other scans intended to investigate setup reproducibility. This data, thus far, have not highlighted any significant differences in position or shape of the patients' treatment volumes, even for the largest breast case.

Two additional CTs were further acquired for the first ten patients during the course of treatment, approximately after 36 Gy (RBE) (20 fractions) and 46.8 Gy (RBE) (26 fractions), respectively. These CT scans were then rigidly registered to the planning CT in order to assess potential swelling. The registration was based on the breast surface and external BB markers, rather than the bony anatomy over the whole CT volume. The rationale for such registration technique is that it corresponds to what is performed at the time of setup prior to beam delivery using the surface imaging system (cf Sect. 8.6). An example of such registration is given in Fig. 8.13 for the largest intact breast patient treated. The rescan was acquired after the 26th fraction and shows minimal differences. This work highlighted the surprising lack of swelling for intact breast patients at the end of their treatment using PBS, contrasting to what has been observed with conventional photon delivery techniques. As with adaptive planning for other disease sites, this type of rigorous re-imaging or the use of cone beam CT may be favored for initial cases at new proton centers. As further experience is gained, this may be deemed unnecessary.

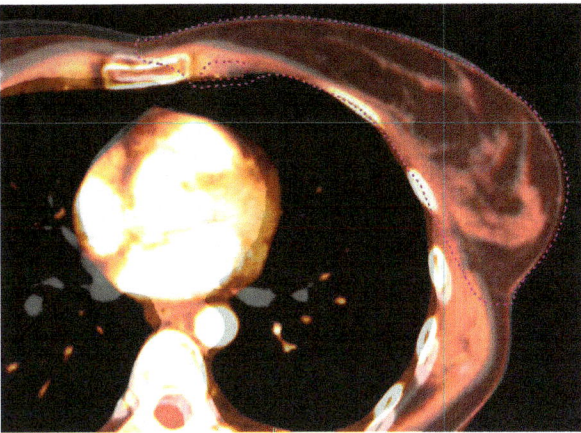

Fig. 8.13 "Surface imaging" registration of the original planning CT scan [red overlay] with a rescan CT acquired toward the end of treatment (26 out of 28 fractions) for the largest intact breast patient treated

8.6 Patient Positioning

Traditionally, patient setup for proton beam treatments relied on X-ray radiographs. The patient is first positioned using tattoos and lasers. A set of orthogonal X-rays is then taken at a cardinal gantry angle to verify the patient's body posture and to place the patient precisely at the isocenter. Finally, a beamline X-ray is performed at the treatment gantry angle to finalize the setup position.

For breast/chest wall treatment, surface imaging may be more representative of the target and more efficient. After initial positioning with lasers and tattoos, a surface image is captured and the calculated position correction applied to our 6-degrees-of-freedom patient positioner (translations and rotations). Multiples iterations may be needed until the position falls below 2 mm and 1°, well within the tolerances derived from MGH-robustness analysis (3 mm/2°). The beamline X-ray image is performed at the end as a final confirmation of the setup [21].

8.6.1 Markers/Region of Interest

For PBS postmastectomy proton radiation therapy (PMRT) patients, six tattoos are inked at the time of CT simulation: three inferior tattoos for leveling, two at the level of the breast (midline and treatment side), and one in the supraclavicular area. These tattoos are used first to position the patient with lasers and second to study potential changes in the shape of the chest. Radio-opaque markers are taped daily on the three upper tattoos and used as a final confirmation of the surface image-based setup.

Surface imaging techniques require a reference surface to which the acquired daily patient surface images are compared. For this reference, one can use a surface image captured at the time of CT simulation (if surface imaging is available in the

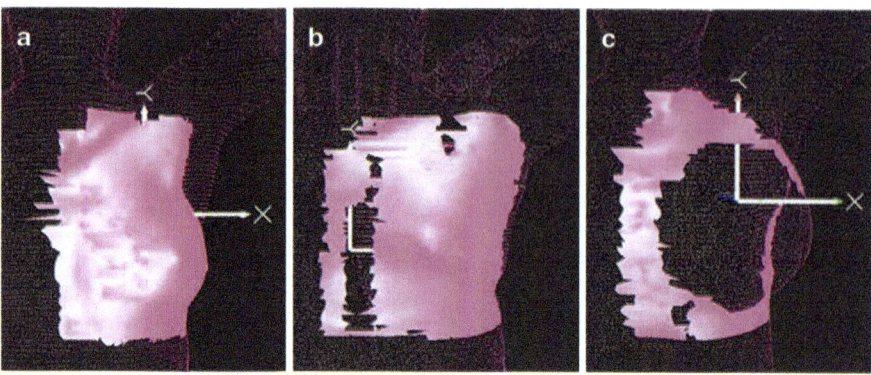

Fig. 8.14 Examples of region of interest for various patient type

room), a surface image captured at the time of treatment, or use the body surface generated from the patient's simulation CT data.

Depending on the patient's target volume, three ROI shapes may be used: chest wall patient with implant ROI including the target volume (chest wall + nodes) and excluding the armpit and the upper node target area (Fig. 8.14a), chest wall patient without implant ROI including the target volume and part of the arm and excluding the upper node target area (Fig. 8.14b), or intact breast patient ROI including the chest wall surrounding the breast tissue and excluding the armpit and the upper node target area (Fig. 8.14c).

8.6.2   Image Acquisition Mode

The AlignRT© surface imaging system developed by Vision RT Ltd (London, UK) allows for three "types" of acquisition: "treatment" images, "gated" images, and "monitoring."

The "treatment" image is a snapshot; the displayed shifts represent the immediate shifts of the patient compared to the reference. In the AlignRT© "gated" mode, the patient's respiratory motion is monitored using a virtual tracking point located near the middle of the abdomen. The monitoring (or real time) display provides immediate feedback on any variation in patient position during the setup.

8.6.3   Surface Imaging Workflow

At the Massachusetts General Hospital, surface imaging is currently employed for proton beam treatment verification. After initial positioning with lasers and tattoos, the first image at gantry 0° is a "treatment" snapshot, and the displayed corrections based on the selected target ROI are applied. A second snapshot image is then acquired in order to verify that the intended corrections were applied and to interactively adjust arm and chin positions. A subsequent set of images are acquired using the "monitoring" mode. Most PBS treatment time does not allow for breath-hold treatments as treatment delivery time is approximately 2 min, thus leaving the patient breathing freely during treatment. Despite the fact that the amplitude of the chest wall motion during quiet respiration is generally small (<3 mm), the "monitoring" mode is used throughout the setup process and allows for therapist to confirm that the patient position remains in tolerance during the breathing cycle.

The gantry is then rotated to the treatment angle (generally 30° or 330°) and the patient position confirmed using surface imaging (monitoring mode) and ultimately X-ray imaging.

All Align RT© images are acquired with the snout retracted to allow the optimal field of view; the snout is therefore sent to the treatment position moments before delivery.

8.6.4   X-Ray Confirmation

A final X-ray image based on three skin markers is performed before treatment. The analysis of ten patients' X-ray images acquired before treatment and after positioning with surface imaging shows a Gaussian distribution of the residual X-ray shifts with 1.1 mm ± 1.2 σ in the lateral direction, -1.0 mm ± 1.2 σ in the longitudinal direction, and -0.6 mm ± 0.7 σ in the vertical direction, as highlighted in Fig. 8.15. These data confirmed the accuracy of the surface imaging positioning.

These residual shifts may be attributed to several factors. For one, the markers represent the positions of only three points on the skin surface, the surface imaging system uses a region of interest that nearly covers the entire chest wall for surface matching. The consistency of the marker positions is also limited by uncertainties at many steps including tattooing, marker placement, and localization of the marker positions due to finite CT slice spacing and artifacts. For these reasons, only half of the magnitude of the marker-based position corrections is applied when outside of the robustness tolerance thresholds (i.e., > 3 mm). These over-tolerance shifts

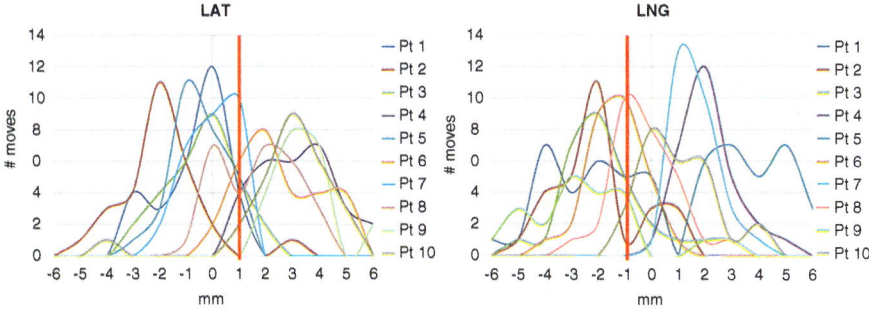

Fig. 8.15 Skin marker X-ray-based shifts after surface image positioning for ten patients. Each point represents the occurrence of shifts during the treatment (28 fractions), the *red line* the average over all

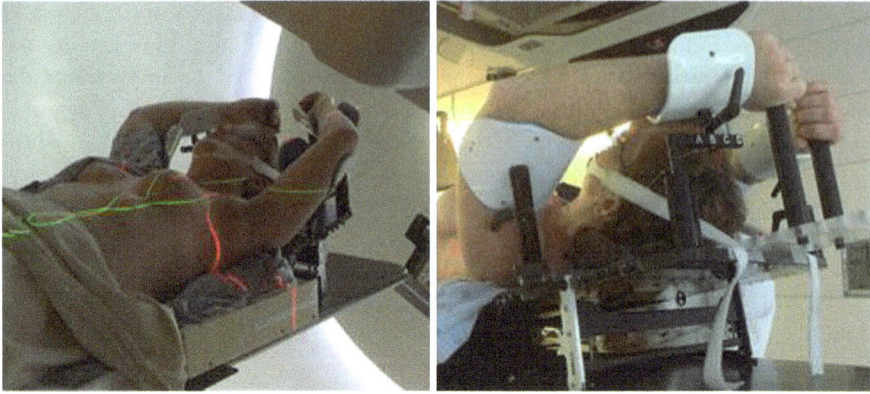

Fig. 8.16 Patient positioned arms-up in the treatment room with the breast board at the highest angle available, head and neck head cup and additional handgrips and chin strap

occurred in the longitudinal and lateral direction for 15 % of the 10 patient's fractions, representing an average of four fractions per patient. Consistently large magnitude shifts, however, may indicate a change in the patient shape (shift of implant, swelling) and result in a new CT acquisition to assess if re-planning is necessary.

The X-ray acquisition also provides an independent check of the surface image isocenter which, in our facility, is entered manually.

8.7   Setup Positions

8.7.1   Arms-Up

PMRT patients are generally positioned on a conventional commercial breast board with both arms up above their head. The board is raised to the highest angle available in order to limit missing data on the surface imaging system at the time of setup. The missing data issue arises on the upper part of the patient's chest due to the suboptimal position of the surface imaging cameras caused by the large gantry rotation structure and lower ceiling.

Since nodal and target volumes are covered using a single PBS field, the chin and arms positions (noted to have more variation on AlignRT©) are of importance for proper delivery. The original soft head rest on the breast board may be replaced by a head and neck head cup to better control the neck position. A chin strap combine with a spirit angle measurement insures the daily chin position. Handgrips may also be added on the original breast board to better maintain arm position. Figure 8.16 offers an overall view of the arms-up setup position.

Figure 8.17 provides examples of patient surface images after positioning based on the setup information compared to the expected treatment position from the planning CT surface.

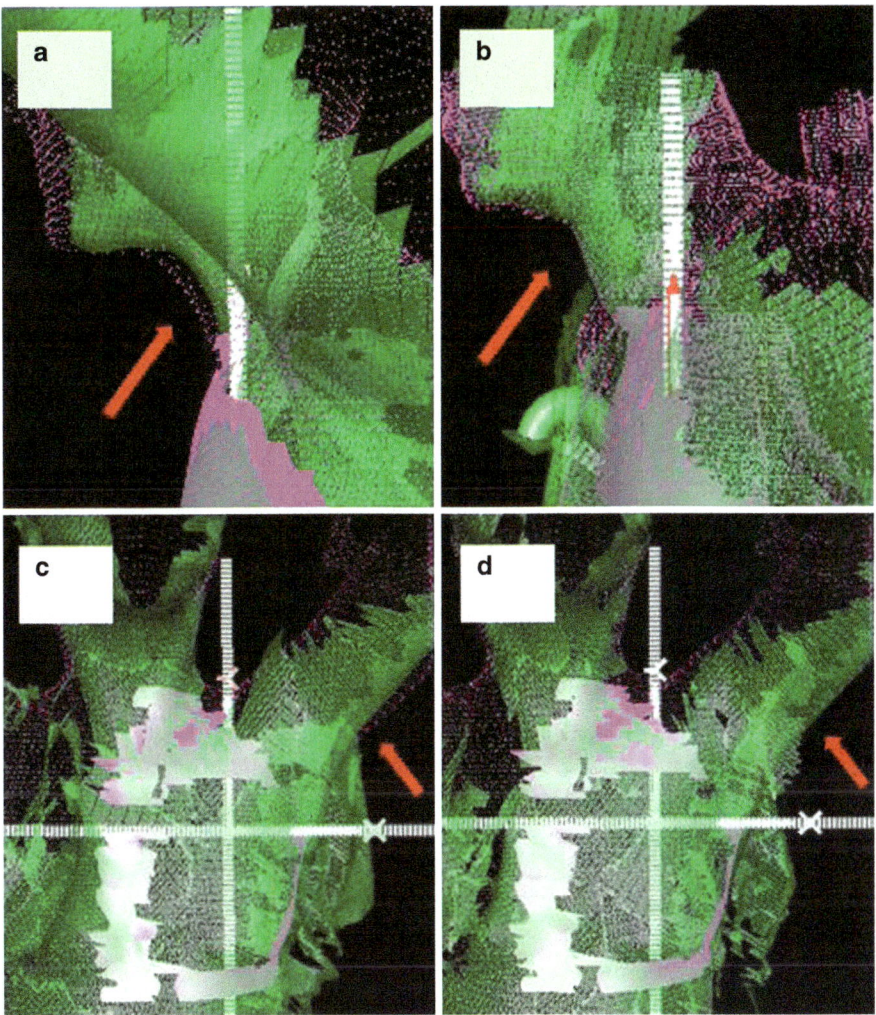

Fig. 8.17 Patient surface image (*green*) overlaid onto the planning CT surface (*pink*); (**a**) error in the head cup, (**b**) expected chin/neck position, (**c**) initial arms position, (**d**) adjusted arm position

8.7.2 Arms-Down

The "en face" beam approach used for proton delivery does not require the traditional arms-up position that is mandatory when using tangents beams. Though traditional positioning is still used for most patients, patients with great difficulty tolerating standard positioning due to the immediacy of the axillary nodal dissection, or other immobility factors, may be treated in a more comfortable "arms-down" position. Contours can be more challenging due to the change in anatomy. The use of a high-angle board allows a posterior-akimbo position with a large

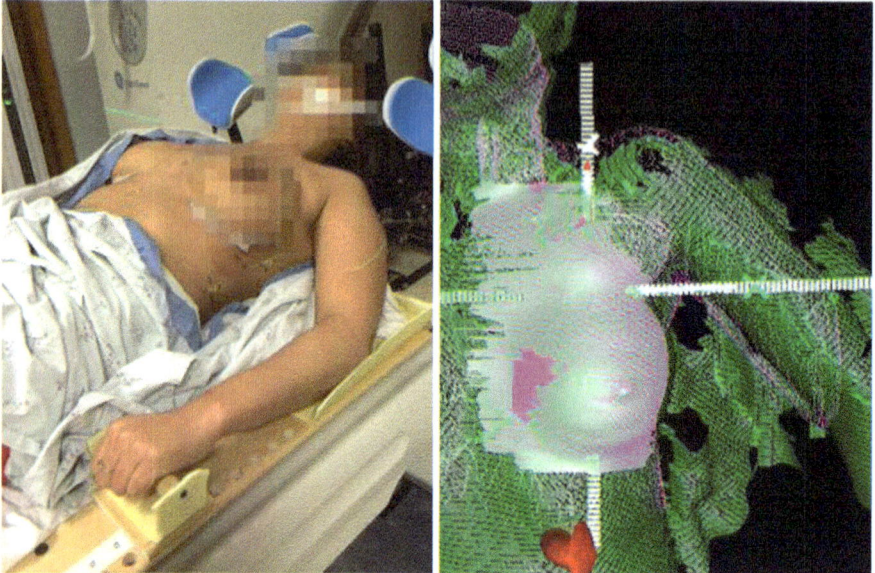

Fig. 8.18 Arms-down posterior-akimbo position with horizontal handgrip and its associated patient surface image

opening of the patient side and underarms. Horizontal handgrips may be designed to reproduce the arm position. An overall view of the arms-down position is given in Fig. 8.18.

8.7.3   Timing/Efficiency

Efficiency may be improved by surface imaging. For AlignRT© positioning, a time stamp records each acquisition along the positioning and treatment processes. These time stamps (in seconds) have been used to estimate the length of each step in the positioning process, as well as the overall time spent by the patient in the room [21]. AlignRT images acquired after initial positioning with laser and tattoos and surface images acquired before treatment give an estimation of the setup time. Surface images acquired before leaving the room (after setup) and re-entering the room after treatment give an estimate of the treatment time. Results showed that the X-ray only setup procedure took 11 min on average, while the surface imaging gated positioning process and the surface imaging monitoring process (after initial positioning with lasers and tattoos) took 6 min and 3 min, respectively (Fig. 8.19). The treatment time – including moving the snout down after surface imaging and up after treatment, therapists exiting and entering the room, and requesting of the beam shared between rooms – was averaging at 5 min, including 2 min beam on time.

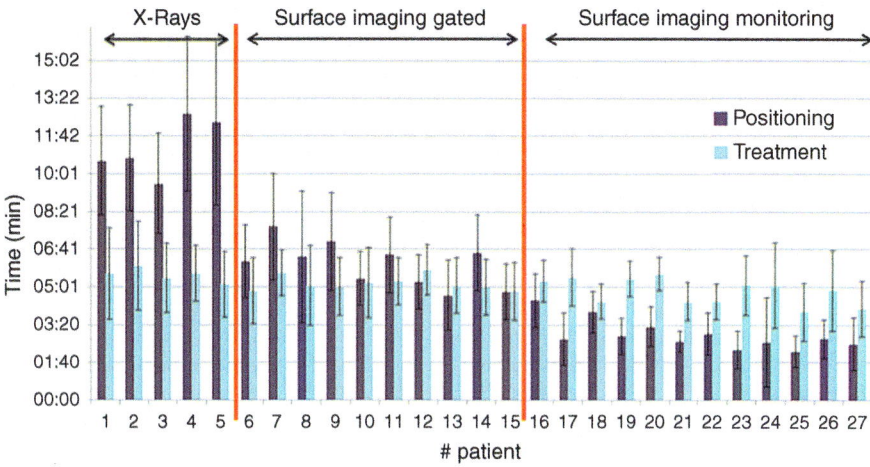

Fig. 8.19 Treatment delivery (*light*) and setup time (*dark*) for an "en face" field positioned with X-rays, gated surface image, or monitoring surface image

Conclusions

At present, the use of proton radiation for breast cancer is still in its infancy [22]. However, its use for the breast cancer population is anticipated to increase rapidly as early experience is published, the number of proton facilities increase, and smaller less costly proton accelerators become available. In time, it is predicted that further advances will allow for costs to decrease and proton therapy to become more widely available [23]. It is even possible that, for some patients with breast cancer, protons may prove to be cost-effective [24]. As this chapter is being written, the first patients are being enrolled on the Patient-Centered Outcomes Research Institute (PCORI) funded Radiotherapy Comparative Effectiveness (RADCOMP) Consortium pragmatic randomized trial of proton therapy versus photon therapy for patients with non-metastatic breast cancer receiving comprehensive nodal radiation including the internal mammary nodes. This trial has 22 participating centers and anticipates additional institutions to join as more proton centers are planned.

References

1. MacDonald SM, Patel SA, Hickey S et al (2013) Proton therapy for breast cancer after mastectomy: early outcomes of a prospective clinical trial. Int J Radiat Oncol Biol Phys 86:484–490
2. Galland-Girodet S, Pashtan I, MacDonald SM et al (2014) Long-term cosmetic outcomes and toxicities of proton beam therapy compared with photon-based 3-dimensional conformal accelerated partial-breast irradiation: a phase 1 trial. Int J Radiat Oncol Biol Phys 90:493–500
3. Cuaron JJ, Chon B, Tsai H et al (2015) Early toxicity in patients treated with postoperative proton therapy for locally advanced breast cancer. Int J Radiat Oncol Biol Phys 92:284–291

4. Lancellotti P, Nkomo VT, Badano LP et al (2013) Expert consensus for multi-modality imaging evaluation of cardiovascular complications of radiotherapy in adults: a report from the European Association of Cardiovascular Imaging and the American Society of Echocardiography. J Am Soc Echocardiogr 26:1013–1032
5. Nilsson G, Holmberg L, Garmo H et al (2012) Distribution of coronary artery stenosis after radiation for breast cancer. J Clin Oncol 30:380–386
6. Darby SC, Ewertz M, McGale P et al (2013) Risk of ischemic heart disease in women after radiotherapy for breast cancer. N Engl J Med 368:987–998
7. MacDonald SM, Jimenez R, Paetzold P et al (2013) Proton radiotherapy for chest wall and regional lymphatic radiation; dose comparisons and treatment delivery. Radiat Oncol 8:71
8. Jimenez RB, Goma C, Nyamwanda J et al (2013) Intensity modulated proton therapy for post-mastectomy radiation of bilateral implant reconstructed breasts: a treatment planning study. Radiother Oncol 107:213–217
9. MacDonald SM, Harisinghani MG, Katkar A et al (2010) Nanoparticle-enhanced MRI to evaluate radiation delivery to the regional lymphatics for patients with breast cancer. Int J Radiat Oncol Biol Phys 77:1098–1104
10. Tepper J, Verhey L, Goitein M et al (1977) In vivo determinations of RBE in a high energy modulated proton beam using normal tissue reactions and fractionated dose schedules. Int J Radiat Oncol Biol Phys 2:1115–1122
11. Paganetti H, Niemierko A, Ancukiewicz M et al (2002) Relative biological effectiveness (RBE) values for proton beam therapy. Int J Radiat Oncol Biol Phys 53:407–421
12. Liss AL, Ben-David MA, Jagsi R et al (2014) Decline of cosmetic outcomes following accelerated partial breast irradiation using intensity modulated radiation therapy: results of a single-institution prospective clinical trial. Int J Radiat Oncol Biol Phys 89:96–102
13. Peterson D, Truong PT, Parpia S et al (2015) Predictors of adverse cosmetic outcome in the RAPID trial: an exploratory analysis. Int J Radiat Oncol Biol Phys 91:968–976
14. Kozak KR, Smith BL, Adams J et al (2006) Accelerated partial-breast irradiation using proton beams: initial clinical experience. Int J Radiat Oncol Biol Phys 66:691–698
15. Bush DA, Slater JD, Garberoglio C et al (2007) A technique of partial breast irradiation utilizing proton beam radiotherapy: comparison with conformal x-ray therapy. Cancer J 13:114–118
16. Bush DA, Slater JD, Garberoglio C et al (2011) Partial breast irradiation delivered with proton beam: results of a phase II trial. Clin Breast Cancer 11:241–245
17. Bush DA, Do S, Lum S et al (2014) Partial breast radiation therapy with proton beam: 5-year results with cosmetic outcomes. Int J Radiat Oncol Biol Phys 90:501–505
18. Wang X, Amos RA, Zhang X et al (2011) External-beam accelerated partial breast irradiation using multiple proton beam configurations. Int J Radiat Oncol Biol Phys 80:1464–1472
19. Ares C, Hug EB, Lomax AJ et al (2009) Effectiveness and safety of spot scanning proton radiation therapy for chordomas and chondrosarcomas of the skull base: first long-term report. Int J Radiat Oncol Biol Phys 75:1111–1118
20. Depauw N, Batin E, Daartz J et al (2015) A novel approach to postmastectomy radiation therapy using scanned proton beams. Int J Radiat Oncol Biol Phys 91:427–434
21. Batin E, Depauw N, MacDonald S et al (2016) Can surface imaging improve the patient setup for proton postmastectomy chest wall irradiation? Pract Radiat Oncol. Feb 13.
22. MacDonald SM (2016) Proton therapy for breast cancer: getting to the heart of the matter. Int J Radiat Oncol Biol Phys 95:46–48
23. Goitein M, Jermann M (2003) The relative costs of proton and X-ray radiation therapy. Clin Oncol 15:S37–S50
24. Mailhot Vega RB, Ishaq O, Raldow A et al (2016) Establishing cost-effective allocation of proton therapy for breast irradiation. Int J Radiat Oncol Biol Phys 95:11–18

Hyperthermia in Locally Recurrent Breast Cancer

9

Tracy Sherertz and Chris J. Diederich

Contents

9.1   Introduction

Locally recurrent breast cancer poses a major therapeutic challenge, especially in a patient who has received prior radiotherapy and treatment options are limited at the time of recurrence. Estimates of locoregional recurrence rates from large randomized trials range from 5 to 15 % of all patients with breast cancer treated with definitive intent postmastectomy or postlumpectomy radiotherapy [1–4]. Of the patients who recur, the ipsilateral breast or chest wall is the most common site of recurrence, representing up to 95 % of all locoregional recurrences [5–7]. Symptoms of a recurrent tumor in the chest wall can be devastating, with profound effects on quality of life. Such symptoms can include intractable pain, bleeding, infection, deformity, impaired breathing from lung invasion, and foul-smelling wounds requiring daily

T. Sherertz, MD (✉)
Department of Radiation Oncology, University of California, San Francisco,
1600 Divisadero St. Ste H1031, San Francisco, CA 94115, USA
e-mail: Tracy.Sherertz@ucsf.edu

C.J. Diederich, PhD
Medical Physics Division, Department of Radiation Oncology,
University of California, San Francisco, San Francisco, CA, USA

© Springer International Publishing Switzerland 2016   145
J.R. Bellon et al. (eds.), *Radiation Therapy Techniques and Treatment Planning
for Breast Cancer*, Practical Guides in Radiation Oncology,
DOI 10.1007/978-3-319-40392-2_9

wound care. Isolated axillary or supraclavicular recurrences are observed less frequently than chest wall recurrences, ranging from 0.5 to 3.0 % [8, 9]; however, these patients also have a 50–65 % risk of developing distant metastatic disease [10, 11]. Given their location, however, axillary and supraclavicular recurrences tend to cause significant morbidity such as pain, lymphedema, impaired range of motion, and brachial plexopathy and may therefore require locoregional treatment despite the competing risk for distant metastases that will be treated with systemic therapy.

Radiation therapy has evolved to play a significant role in the management of locally recurrent disease. When patients recur locally after breast conservation therapy, mastectomy is generally the preferred approach, as these patients have already received a definitive course of radiotherapy, inevitably including some dose to the adjacent normal tissues. Breast cancer that recurs locally following mastectomy in previously irradiated patients, however, poses a greater challenge. Common practice is to initiate systemic therapy in effort to cytoreduce the tumor and thereby minimize the volume of tissue requiring re-irradiation, which is analogous to using neoadjuvant chemotherapy in unresectable disease. When surgery is not a viable option, as in cases where a resection would leave the patient with an unacceptable defect, palliative re-irradiation is generally indicated to enhance local control. Historically, re-irradiation was used with great caution, due to concern for an increased risk for late normal tissue complications. One of the earliest studies to report on re-irradiation in the setting of locally recurrence chest wall disease was by Laramore et al., in which 13 patients were re-irradiated with conventionally fractionated electrons after having received initial chest wall radiotherapy doses of 40–50 Gy. With a median follow-up of only 12 months, eight patients (62 %) were alive and free of local recurrence, and skin reactions ranged from temporary erythema to dry and moist desquamation [12]. Thereafter, several modest-sized clinical trials investigated the use of re-irradiation in the setting of local recurrence, and re-irradiation was reported to cause a < 12 % risk of late grade 3 toxicity, which was considered by many to be acceptable, in light of the lack of other safe treatment options [5, 12–16].

9.2   Background of Hyperthermia

Re-irradiation is now regarded as potentially safe with careful dose composite calculations to normal tissues, yet the re-irradiation dose can be severely limited due to concerns for normal tissue toxicity. The lower the re-irradiation dose, the safer the treatment, but the tumor control probability also decreases. Hyperthermia, treatment at elevated temperatures, was therefore investigated as an adjunct modality to radiotherapy in the 1970s and 1980s, because it was known to cause complementary effects in cells when combined with radiotherapy. At the cellular level, heat causes damage to DNA, proteins, and cell membranes, interferes with the cell cycle, and impairs DNA and protein synthesis, thereby impairing DNA damage repair which will lead to cell death either directly or via apoptosis [17]. Multiple mechanisms of action have been reported on the combined effectiveness of radiotherapy and hyperthermia, including direct thermal cytotoxicity of necrotic, hypoxic, and nutritionally deprived cells, denaturing proteins which will prevent repair of sublethal and potentially lethal DNA damage, and changes in tissue perfusion which increases tumor oxygenation and results in radiosensitization [18, 19]. The downstream effects of hyperthermia, including reoxygenation, have been shown to be sustainable for greater than 24–48 h for subsequent RT fractions [20].

With the goal of optimizing local control, especially when re-irradiation doses are limited by a patient's prior RT dose, hyperthermia was combined with re-irradiation in multiple early studies that subsequently illuminated the benefit and toxicities of this combined approach (Table 9.1). Five studies addressing the effect of adding hyperthermia to radiation for superficial localized breast cancer were initiated between 1988 and 1991. Unfortunately, these studies suffered from slow recruitment and lack of consistent goals for target temperatures. This led to a decision to collaborate and combine the trial results into one analysis and report them simultaneously in one publication [27]. Of the 306 patients randomized, the overall complete response rate for RT alone was 41 % versus 59 % for RT + HT group, with the caveat that not all of the trials demonstrated an advantage for the combined treatment. Despite the methodological limitations of this combined analysis, the greatest effect was observed in patients who recurred in previously irradiated areas. Toxicity across the five trials was not consistently reported; however, of the available data, the incidence of mild/moderate erythema, severe erythema, telangiectasia, and hyperpigmentation was equal across the RT and RT/HT arms. Blistering was slightly more common in the combined RT/HT arms compared to the RT alone arms, 11 % versus 2 %, respectively, but this increase was noted in four out of the five trials. Ulceration and necrosis were also slightly more common in the RT/HT arms compared to the RT alone arms, 7 % versus 2 % (ulceration) and 7 % versus 1 % (necrosis). Severe late toxicities occurred in only one of the trials, European Society for Hyperthermic Oncology; out of the 56 patients on this trial, there was one case of bone necrosis, one case of bone fracture, and one brachial plexus toxicity all of which occurred in the combined RT/HT arm. Data on total composite dose to critical structures are not available; however at least 22 patients across all trials were treated to a nodal volume that included the brachial plexus. With only one reported brachial plexopathy reported, HT as delivered in these trials was well tolerated and did not appear to significantly add to the acute or late toxicity associated with re-irradiation.

In a more recent trial published in 2005, Jones et al. conducted a prospective randomized study of superficial recurrent tumors (<3 cm depth) comparing radiotherapy versus radiotherapy + hyperthermia [22]. One hundred twenty-two patients were enrolled; 109 (89 %) were deemed eligible for hyperthermia and 70 of these were patients with breast cancer. The investigators were among the first to carefully incorporate a highly controlled thermal dose prescription and administration. They used the parameter describing the number of cumulative minutes at 43 °C exceeded by 90 % of monitored points within the tumor (CEM 43 °C T_{90}) as a measure of thermal dose. The complete response rate was 66.1 % in the RT + HT arm versus

Table 9.1 Outcomes reported following re-irradiation +/− hyperthermia

Author	Study design	n	Follow-up	Initial RT dose (Gy)	Technique	Re-RT dose	% complete response (in-field)	% grade 3 toxicity	% grade 4 toxicity
Laramore [12]	Retrospective	13	9 months to 5 years	40–50	EBRT	40–50	61.5 %	0	0
Phromratanapongse [14]	Retrospective	44	1 month	35–66	EBRT+HT	16–56	40.9	25	–
Li [21]	Retrospective	41	6 months	58	EBRT+HT	43±12.4 Gy	56	–	8
Jones [22]	Prospective, randomized	52 56	2–9 years	NR (17 had prior RT) NR (22 had prior RT)	EBRT EBRT+HT	60–70 30–66	42.3 66.1	2 3	–
Kouloulias [23]	Prospective, phase I/II	15	Median 4 months	60	EBRT+HT *concurrent liposomal doxorubicin	30.6	20	–	7
Zagar [24]	Retrospective	27	11 months	60.4	EBRT+HT+chemo	Median 45	80	0.7	0
Linthorst [16] *post-resection(*)	Retrospective	198	Median 42 months	48	EBRT+HT	32	78	11.9 % (grade 3 or 4)	0
Linthorst [25] *unresectable	Retrospective	248	Median 32 months	49	EBRT+HT	32	70 (<1 year) 53 (1 year) 40 (3 years) 39 (5 years)	1 (at 5 years)	0
Oldenborg [26] *post-resection or chemo	Retrospective	78	Median 64.2 months	≥50	EBRT+HT	32	78 (3 years) 65 (5 years)	32 % (acute grade 3)	40 % after 3 years (grade 3/4)

42.3 % in the irradiation alone arm ($p = 0.02$). Previously irradiated patients had the greatest incremental gain in complete response: 23.5 % in the irradiation alone arm versus 68.2 % in the RT + HT arm. There was no observed benefit in overall survival [22]. Side effects were mostly limited to grade 1 and 2 acute skin toxicity. Grade 1 skin toxicity was noted in 25 % of patients in the RT/HT arm versus 4 % in the arm without hyperthermia; grade 2 toxicity was noted in 16 % of patients receiving RT/HT versus 0 % in the RT alone arm. Grade 3 skin toxicity was noted in 5 % of the RT/HT arm and 2 % of the RT alone arm.

Many patients with locoregional recurrences receive concurrent systemic therapies in order to treat simultaneous distant recurrences. Historically there has been concern over the combined toxicity risk when chemotherapy, radiotherapy, and hyperthermia are all delivered concurrently. Recently, a small retrospective series was published on the potential benefit and additional toxicities of treating chest wall recurrences with a combination of all three modalities. Zagar et al. reported on 27 patients with chest wall recurrences from breast cancer treated with concurrent superficial twice-weekly hyperthermia, radiotherapy, and systemic chemotherapy (capecitabine in 21, vinorelbine in 2, and paclitaxel in 4). With a median follow-up of 11 months, there was an 80 % complete clinical response rate. Overall survival was 23 months for those patients with a complete response versus only 5.4 months for patients achieving only a partial response. Eighty-one percent of patients experienced a grade 1 or 2 acute skin toxicity, with two patients experiencing grade 3 toxicity, both resolving with conservative measure [24]. Prospective data are still lacking for outcomes from concurrent combination of all three modalities.

Phase I data have recently been reported using low-temperature liposomal doxorubicin (LTLD) combined with local hyperthermia in heavily pretreated patients with locoregionally recurrent breast cancer [28]. In two similarly designed phase 1 trials, 29 patients received 6 cycles of LTLD every 21–35 days followed immediately by chest wall hyperthermia for 1 h at 40–42 °C. The maximum tolerated dose of LDTD was 50 mg/m^2, and seven patients (24 %) developed reversible grade 3–4 neutropenia and four patients (14 %) developed reversible leucopenia. Overall local response rate (in the HT field) was 48 % (14/29 patients) with five patients (17 %) achieving a complete local response and nine patients (31 %) achieving a partial response. Prospective data in larger patient cohorts are still lacking. In general, chemotherapy with HT would be preferable for heavily pretreated patients with multiple or symptomatic sites of metastatic disease who are responding well to chemotherapy at distant sites but not responding well at the local recurrence. In patients where local control becomes the primary concern, however, RT + HT would be preferable. This is also true when patients reach a point where they can no longer tolerate systemic therapy and are interested in local palliation of a recurrent lesion.

Clinical hyperthermia systems are now generally used to heat a tumor target region to approximately 39.5–45 °C for 30–60 min either immediately before or after a radiation fraction [29–31]. A typical palliative re-irradiation dose used with hyperthermia is 400 cGy delivered twice weekly for a total of eight fractions to a

Large central necrotic mass   Nodular diffuse recurrence that
not responsive to chemo   progressed through chemo

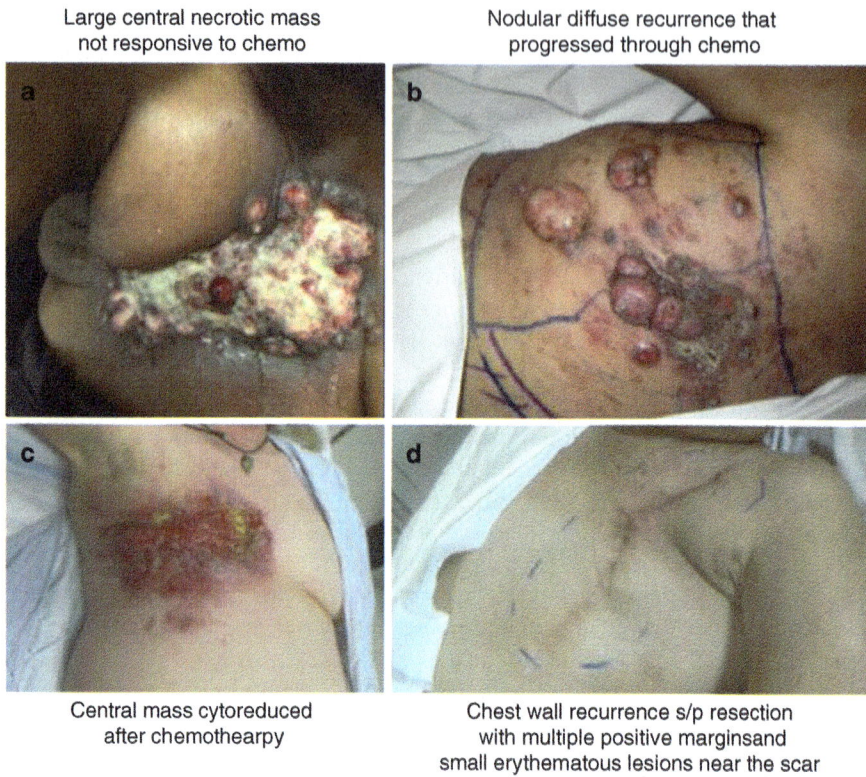

Central mass cytoreduced   Chest wall recurrence s/p resection
after chemothearpy   with multiple positive marginsand
                                             small erythematous lesions near the scar

Fig. 9.1 Range of locally recurrent breast cancer cases treated with radiation and hyperthermia. (**a**) Large central necrotic mass not responsive to chemo. (**b**) Nodular diffuse recurrence that progressed through chemo. (**c**) Central mass cytoreduced after chemotherapy. (**d**) Chest wall recurrence s/p resection with multiple positive margins and small erythematous lesions near the scar

dose of 32 Gy. Hyperthermia can also be combined with other fractionation schemes to augment RT in any situation where recurrent disease is being treated. Re-irradiation doses and fractionation schemes will be dictated by a patient's prior RT dose.

Figure 9.1 shows the spectrum of the types of locoregional recurrences from breast cancer that have been treated with RT and hyperthermia, ranging from erythematous skin changes only, to more bulky nodular type of chest wall recurrences.

9.3 Delivery of Hyperthermia

Hyperthermia can be delivered to tumors externally using superficially positioned devices, as well as internally via body cavities and interstitial implants [32, 33]. The most common energy modalities to generate heat therapy are electromagnetic (EM) and ultrasound technologies and are most applicable to the external superficial treatment of recurrent breast cancer. The EM microwave systems in general consist of a waveguide(s) operating at 434 MHz (Europe & Asia) or 915 MHz (USA), coupled by an air gap or a temperature-regulated water bolus, which is placed directly over the target and can heat up to 1–4 cm deep. The temperature of the water coupling can be regulated to control the temperature of the skin and push the maximum temperature deeper in the tissue. Guidelines specific to each type of MW waveguide and system need to be followed, ensuring that the effective power deposition pattern encompasses the target volume. The effective therapeutic zones of microwave applicators range from 2 to 3 cm diameter to greater than 20 cm × 30 cm, with some devices capable of conforming to the chest wall contour. Ultrasound systems [34] consist of large and small superficial multielement devices that can cover 15 cm × 15 cm area or 7.5 cm × 7.5 cm area, respectively, with integrated water coupling. The frequency of operation can be selected to 3.4 MHz for heating up to ~4 cm depth, and 1 MHz to extend heating up to 8 cm deep from the surface.

Both ultrasound- and microwave-based modalities are sensitive to tissue heterogeneity (i.e., bone vs. muscle) as well as spatial and dynamic changes in blood flow. Delivery of a fairly uniform temperature distribution within the tumor volume is important to minimize the risk of thermal damage and also to ensure optimal therapeutic benefit. Safe hyperthermia delivery requires careful monitoring of the surface temperatures by placing thermometry probes on the target surface throughout the hyperthermia. For superficial disease extending less than 1 cm depth from the skin, surface temperature sensors only are typically used; for deeper targets greater than 1 cm depth, invasive needle temperature probes can be placed within the tumor at depth. Inevitably, nodular recurrences where the target surface is not flat or of uniform thickness pose a challenge, so it may be necessary to use both surface thermometry for regions < 1 cm thick and needle temperature probes for areas of tumor > 1 cm thick. The planning CT simulation scan is used to determine depth. Temperature sensing is critical for controlling the delivery of hyperthermia and calculating the thermal dose. Control of the applicator power levels, positioning of the applicator, and water bolus temperature can be adjusted to best provide therapeutic temperatures. The conventional objective is to initiate hyperthermia within 30–60 min of a radiation fraction and treat for a duration of 60 min with a goal of obtaining a minimum thermal dose of 6–10 CEM 43 °C in greater than 90 % of the monitored points within the tumor [22]. When treating twice weekly, hyperthermia is delivered with each radiotherapy fraction. When treating with 180–200 cGy per fraction, hyperthermia is usually delivered twice weekly, not daily with each fraction.

The appropriate hyperthermia device can be selected to heat the specific target, whether it is superficial microscopic disease or large diffuse areas of chest wall recurrence, intact breast, and axillary or supraclavicular disease. The depth of the target, as in the case with unresectable axillary or supraclavicular disease, will help dictate the most appropriate hyperthermia device to use. For example, ultrasound systems can generally provide deeper penetration of heat than microwave-based systems. Tumor and tissue heterogeneity is another important consideration, whereas blood flow changes, tissue layers, convex geometry, or variable tumor thickness across the target need to be accommodated in treatment. For example, as energy and heat will not penetrate effectively through the bone, tumor lying beneath the bone, such as the sternum, will likely not be adequately heated by superficial applicators to therapeutic temperatures. Size of the target is another limitation to consider if the target size is larger than the effective heating area of the hyperthermia applicator. In these cases various delivery options exist including the following: the applicator(s) can be applied to separate regions of the target for 30–60 min at a time, possibly before and after the radiation fraction for more extensive disease, so depending on the size of the target, a hyperthermia session could last up to 2–4 h in total duration; alternatively, a dominant or most problematic or bulky region(s) can be defined, targeted, and treated on alternate sessions/days. Since many patients with extensive disease cannot tolerate such a prolonged treatment time, it is often necessary to prioritize heating only the most problematic areas with hyperthermia, such as the portion of the tumor causing pain, ulceration, necrosis, or bleeding.

Requirements for strict immobilization and reproducibility during hyperthermia are not as stringent as they are during delivery of radiation therapy. Patients are typically positioned on a gurney or bed with padding, and pillows and other cushion devices can be used to allow the room for the hyperthermia applicator access to the target and also to optimize patient comfort. If a patient is in pain and requires a small adjustment in their positioning, this can be accomplished during hyperthermia without as much concern about setup as there is when delivering radiation therapy.

Equipment and staffing considerations for a hyperthermia clinic can be found in Myerson et al. [35], and importantly, dedication from an experienced medical physicist is necessary for implementation and quality assurance of the hyperthermia program. Examples of setup and delivery of superficial hyperthermia are shown in Fig. 9.2. Grids are often used to subdivide a large surface target into smaller regions that can each be monitored and labeled consistently at subsequent fractions to ensure temperature sensing throughout the entire target field. Currently, clinical hyperthermia programs exist primarily at only a limited number of high-volume, multidisciplinary cancer centers throughout North America and Europe.

9.4   Skincare for Radiation with Hyperthermia

Wound care is an integral part of caring for patients undergoing re-irradiation, regardless of whether or not delivered with hyperthermia. Daily skin care interventions will be determined by the severity of the skin involvement from tumor as well as severity of skin toxicity due to treatments. Patients with recurrent chest wall tumors often have impaired wound healing due to prior radiotherapy, which can complicate their tolerance of re-irradiation and hyperthermia. In general, a daily mild enzymatic wound cleanser such as Skintegrity™ is used to promote gentle exfoliation. This allows moisturizers better access to penetrate the skin. Moisturizers such as Aquaphor™, calendula, vitamin A&D ointment, or manuka honey are often used. Covering the moisturized wound with a dressing such as a soft silicone (i.e., Mepilex™) or hydrogel colloidal sheet can help prevent friction when other skin is in apposition to the wound. Lastly, early identification and treatment of superficial infections are critical.

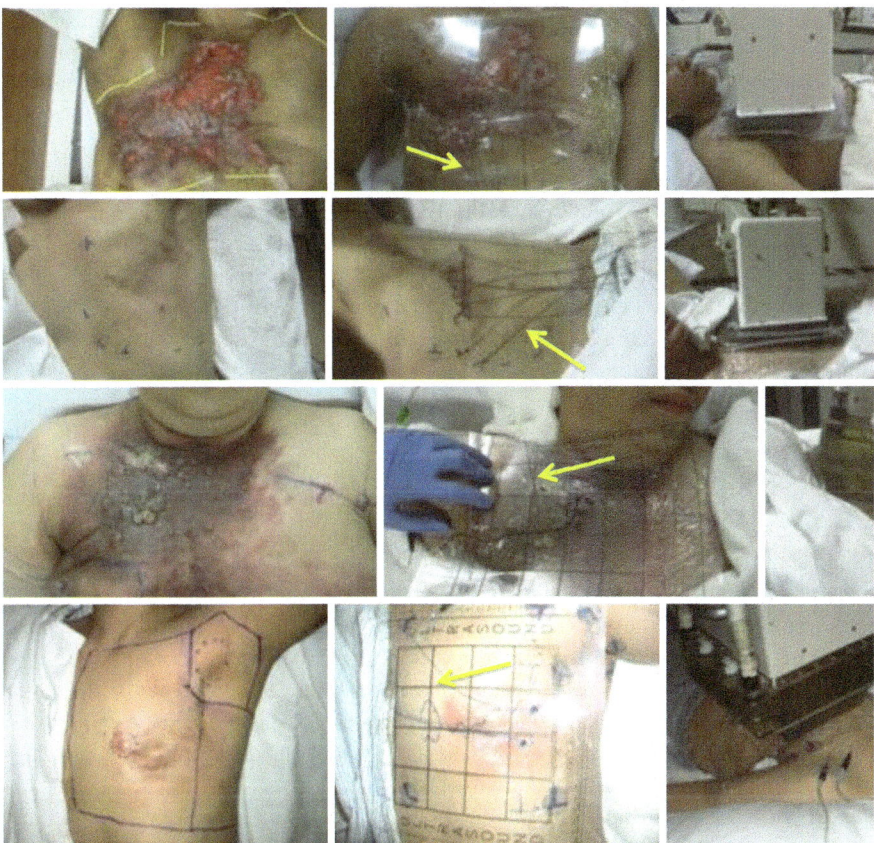

Fig. 9.2 Examples of hyperthermia cases with target site definition (*left*), procedures setup of thermometry sensors beneath applicator layout or template (*middle*, *arrow pointing to sensors*), application for microwave (*top two rows*) and ultrasound hyperthermia (*bottom two rows*) (*right*)

Using metronidazole spray or sprinkling crushed metronidazole onto fungating skin wounds and/or those with a foul smell will help to treat superficial infections and minimize unnecessary irritation of the skin. In the case of moist desquamation, a topical antimicrobial such as zinc, bacitracin, or silvadene is applied to the wound, again dressed with a soft absorbent silicone like Mepilex™, leaving the dressing in place for up to 24 h to minimize trauma to the wound. Cleansing the wound at least once daily with Skintegrity™ or 0.5 Hibiclens™, for example, is recommended.

9.5   Patient Selection

In general, patients with recurrent advanced aggressive disease who have not received prior radiotherapy are recommended to undergo multimodality therapy with radiotherapy, usually without concurrent hyperthermia, allowing for treatment closer to home rather than referral to a high-volume center with a hyperthermia program. But in cases of locally recurrent breast cancer in patients who have received prior irradiation, consideration should be made to add concurrent hyperthermia. The extent of local disease (i.e., macroscopic vs. microscopic, size, depth), presence of controlled concurrent metastases, and patient performance status and goals of care all play into the patient selection criteria. Cytoreduction with chemotherapy prior to radiotherapy is preferable, as this can often reduce the target volume size and minimize the extent of normal tissues in the re-irradiation field. After cytoreduction, usually only the residual measurable disease plus margin is included in the re-irradiated and heated volume. If a patient has already received two prior courses of radiotherapy, re-irradiation is generally not advised, although hyperthermia could be considered as concurrent treatment to systemic chemotherapy. Hyperthermia alone, without concurrent radiotherapy or chemotherapy, is generally not recommended as there is no clear evidence that it provides tumor control benefit as a single modality.

Many patients with recurrent chest wall disease also have distant metastases. The presence of disease outside the radiation treatment area has been observed to have a negative effect on the likelihood of achieving complete response in the treatment field. In the combined analysis of Vernon et al., it was observed that 39% of patients with metastatic disease outside the radiation treatment area achieved a CR in the treatment field, versus 63% for those patients without metastatic disease outside the treated area [27]. This observation could be due to the competing risk of death from progressive disease elsewhere, in which case the patients may not be alive long enough for the tumor in the radiated area to respond completely or be assessed. It is important to note that a complete local control rate of 39% for patients with metastatic disease may still be significant enough to warrant palliation, especially if the distant metastatic disease was treated and/or showing no signs of progression. Thus, the radiation oncologist must carefully assess whether or not the patient can tolerate the prolonged treatment times associated with larger recurrent lesions and also to clarify with patients whether the goal of local control is meaningful in the presence of coexistent metastatic disease.

Based on two large retrospective studies in which patient's tumors were cytoreduced to microscopic disease by either surgery or systemic therapy, it is expected that there will be an improved local control following re-irradiation and hyperthermia, compared to those patient with gross residual or unresectable disease [16, 26]. Linthorst et al. (n=198 patients) and Oldenborg et al. (n=78 patients) reported complete response rates of 78% at approximately 3 years follow-up for patients with microscopic disease only at the time of re-irradiation and hyperthermia. In contrast, the recent report from Linthorst et al. provides an estimate of benefit when delivering re-irradiation with concurrent hyperthermia to patients with gross disease. At 1, 3, and 5 years, the local control was 53, 40, and 39%. The OS in this series declined with longer follow-up: 66% at 1 year, 32% at 3 years, and 18% at 5 years, respectively. Long-term local control, however, was achieved for the 10% of patients alive at 10 years. The incidence of 5-year late grade 3 toxicity in this series was only 1% [25]. This series suggests that the combination of re-irradiation and hyperthermia, even for patients with gross unresectable disease, can result in a high rate of long-term local control with acceptable late toxicity. It is noteworthy that many patients remained locally controlled for the remainder of their lives.

In a recent Dutch analysis of 414 patients treated with re-irradiation and hyperthermia, it was revealed that the size of gross residual disease was a predictor for local recurrence [36]. Compared to tumors <3 cm in size, the hazard ratio for local control steadily increased to 1.6, 2.1, and 2.4 for tumors 3–5 cm, 5–10 cm, and >10 cm, respectively. This report highlights the importance of early referral for patients progressing through systemic therapy and initiation of re-irradiation and hyperthermia for tumors <3 cm, especially in the absence of distant metastases, in order to provide the best chance for local control [36]. In reality though, many patients with recurrence chest wall disease are those patients with rapid progression through systemic therapy, poor access to care, or neglected breast cancers, and these patients may benefit from palliative re-irradiation nevertheless.

In the Phromratanapongse series, tumors heated to a mean thermal dose (equivalent minutes at 42.5 °C) greater than 50 had a 53 % complete response (CR) rate, significantly better than the 14 % CR rate observed in patients whose tumors received a mean thermal dose less than 50 [14]. Among patients with tumors less than or equal to 6 cm^2 in area, 65 % achieved CR, significantly better than the 26 % CR rate noted for patients with tumors greater than 6 cm^2 in area [14]. Similarly, in the combined analysis by Vernon et al., larger tumor size predicted for a decreased chance for achieving complete response [27]. Univariate analysis of the effects of baseline patient characteristics on the CR rate showed that it was strongly dependent on tumor size and depth: CR was achieved in 70 % of patients with tumor area <16 cm^2 versus 45 % for patients whose tumors were ≥16 cm^2, and CR was achieved in 60 % of tumors <3 cm^2 versus 38 % for tumors ≥3 cm^2 [27].

Figure 9.3 shows two examples of patients with very different chest wall recurrences before, during, and 6 weeks after RT/HT. Both patients had received previous

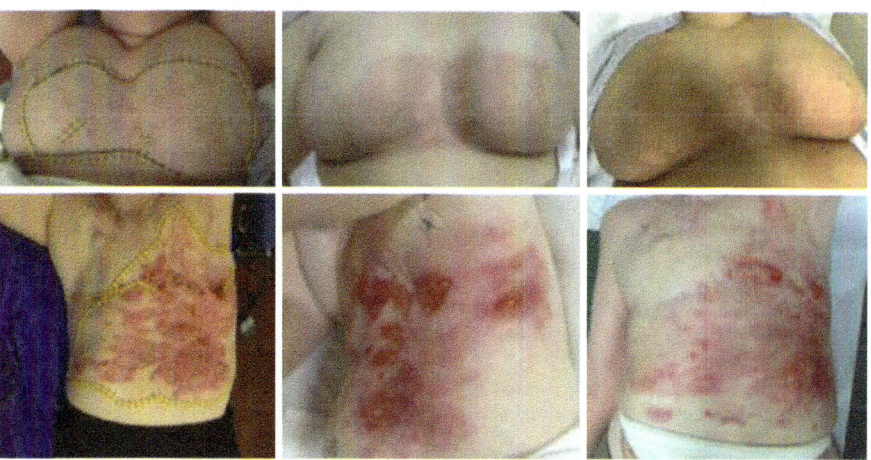

Fig. 9.3 *Top panel*: patient with superficial skin recurrence without distant metastases. Pretreatment photo (*left*), mid-RT/HT photo (*center*), 6-week post-RT/HT photo (*right*). *Bottom panel*: patient with plaque-like thick nodular chest wall recurrence from triple-negative breast cancer who progressed through chemotherapy. Pretreatment photo (*left*), mid-RT/HT photo (*center*), 6-week post-RT/HT photo (*right*)

radiation therapy to a total dose of 60–64 Gy. The patient in the top panel developed a local superficial skin recurrence in the medial chest wall without any distant metastases. The second patient had a triple-negative breast cancer that progressed rapidly despite multiple chemotherapy regimens; she presented from the community with a significant pain from a plaque-like thick nodular recurrence extensively involving her left chest wall and extending onto the right. Both patients were treated with 32 Gy over eight fractions delivered twice weekly with concurrent hyperthermia.

Conclusion

In recurrent breast cancer cases, especially in the setting of re-irradiation, hyperthermia can be used in combination with radiation therapy to improve local tumor control. Complete response within the treatment field has ranged from 20 to 80%, depending on the initial tumor volume being treated. For tumor areas <16 cm^2, local control is expected to be around 70%, versus 45% for patients whose tumors are ≥16 cm^2 [27]. Similarly for tumors <3 cm^2 in depth, local control is expected to be 60% versus 38% for tumors ≥3 cm^2 [27]. In re-irradiated patients, rates of grade 3 toxicity range from 0 to 40% and are expected to be secondary to the re-irradiation dose and fraction size, rather than effects of adding hyperthermia. Patients with uncontrolled metastatic disease have a high competing risk of death, so re-irradiation with hyperthermia is generally reserved for those patients whose metastatic disease has responded to systemic therapy but have persistent local disease. As more advanced image-guided and delivery techniques are increasing the accessibility, safety, and popularity of re-irradiation with concurrent hyperthermia has become a more acceptable method to optimize local control in breast cancer patients with locoregional recurrences.

References

1. Early Breast Cancer Trialists' Collaborative Group (EBCTCG) (2011) Effect of radiotherapy after breast-conserving surgery on 10-year recurrence and 15-year breast cancer death: meta-analysis of individual patient data for 10,801 women in 17 randomised trials. Lancet 378: 1707–1716
2. Early Breast Cancer Trialists' Collaborative Group (EBCTCG) (2014) Effect of radiotherapy after mastectomy and axillary surgery on 10-year recurrence and 20-year breast cancer mortality: meta-analysis of individual patient data for 8135 women in 22 randomised trials. Lancet 383:2127–2135
3. Christiansen P, Al Suliman N, Bjerre K, Moller S (2008) Recurrence pattern and prognosis in low-risk breast cancer patients–data from the DBCG 89-A programme. Acta Oncol 47: 691–703
4. Bartelink H, Maingon P, Poortmans P et al (2015) Whole-breast irradiation with or without a boost for patients treated with breast- conserving surgery for early breast cancer: 20-year follow-up of a randomised phase 3 trial. Lancet Oncol 16:47–56
5. Wahl AO, Rademaker A, Kiel K et al (2008) Multi-institutional review of repeat irradiation of chest wall and breast for recurrent breast cancer. Int J Radiat Oncol Biol Phys 70:477–484

6. Nielsen HM, Overgaard M, Grau C et al (2006) Study of failure pattern among high-risk breast cancer patients with or without post- mastectomy radiotherapy in addition to adjuvant systemic therapy: long term results from the Danish Breast Cancer Co-operative Group DBCG 82b and c randomized studies. J Clin Oncol 24:2268–2275

7. Fourquet A, Campana F, Zafrani B et al (1989) Prognostic factors of breast recurrence in the conservative management of early breast cancer: a 25-year follow-up. Int J Radiat Oncol Biol Phys 17:719–725

8. Voogd AC, Cranenbroek S, de Boer R et al (2005) MJC long-term prognosis of patients with axillary recurrence after axillary dissection for invasive breast cancer. Eur J Surg Oncol 31:485–489

9. Harris EE, Hwang WT, Seyednejad F, Solin LJ (2003) Prognosis after regional lymph node recurrence in patients with stage I–II breast carcinoma treated with breast conservation therapy. Cancer 98:2144–2151

10. Newman LA, Hunt KK, Buchholz T et al (2000) Presentation, management and outcome of axillary recurrence from breast cancer. Am J Surg 180:252–256

11. Van der Sangen MJC, Coebergh JWW, Roumen RMH et al (2003) Detection, treatment, and outcome of isolated supraclavicular recurrence in 42 patients with invasive breast carcinoma. Cancer 98:11–17

12. Laramore GE, Griffin TW, Parker RG, Gerdes AJ (1978) The use of electron beams in treating local recurrence of breast cancer in previously irradiated fields. Cancer 41:991–995

13. Elkort RJ, Kelly W, Mozden PJ, Feldman MI (1980) A combined treatment program for the management of locally recurrent breast cancer following chest wall irradiation. Cancer 46: 647–653

14. Phromratanapongse P, Steeves RA, Severson SB, Paliwal BR (1991) Hyperthermia and irradiation for locally recurrent previously irradiated breast cancer. Strahlenther Onkol 167: 93–97

15. Van der Zee J, van der Holt B, Rietveld PJM et al (1999) Reirradiation combined with hyperthermia in recurrent breast cancer is a worthwhile local palliation. Br J Cancer 79:483–490

16. Linthorst M, van Geel AN, Baaijens M et al (2013) Re-irradiation and hyperthermia after surgery for recurrent breast cancer. Radiother Oncol 109:188–193

17. Oei A, Vriend L, Creezee J et al (2015) Effects of hyperthermia on DNA repair pathways: one treatment to inhibit them all. Radiat Oncol 10:165

18. Kampinga HH (2006) Cell biological effects of hyperthermia alone or combined with radiation or drugs: a short introduction to newcomers in the field. Int J Hyperthermia 22(3):191–196

19. Kampinga HH, Dikomey E (2001) Hyperthermic radiosensitization: mode of action and clinical relevance. Int J Radiat Biol 77(4):399–408

20. Vujaskovic Z, Rosen EL, Blackwell KL et al (2003) Ultrasound guided pO2 measurement of breast cancer reoxygenation after neoadjuvant chemotherapy and hyperthermia treatment. Int J Hyperthermia 19(5):498–506

21. Li G, Mitsumori M, Ogura M et al (2004) Local hyperthermia combined with external irradiation for regional recurrent breast carcinoma. Int J Clin Oncol 9:179–183

22. Jones EL, Oleson JR, Prosnitz LR et al (2005) Randomized trial of hyperthermia and radiation for superficial tumors. J Clin Oncol 23:3079–3085

23. Kouloulias VE, Dardoufas CE, Kouvaris JR et al (2002) Liposomal Doxorubicin in conjunction with re-irradiation and local hyperthermia treatment in recurrent breast cancer: a phase I/II trial. Clin Cancer Res 8:374–382

24. Zagar TM, Higgins KA, Miles EF et al (2010) Durable palliation of breast cancer chest wall recurrence with radiation therapy, hyperthermia, and chemotherapy. Radiother Oncol 97(3):535–540

25. Linthorst M, Baaijens M, Wiggenraad R et al (2015) Local control rate after the combination of re-irradiation and hyperthermia for irresectable recurrent breast cancer: Results in 248 patients. Radiother Oncol 117:217–222

26. Oldenborg S, Van Os RM, Van rij CM et al (2010) Elective re-irradiation and hyperthermia following resection of persistent locoregional recurrent breast cancer: a retrospective study. Int J Hyperthermia 26(2):136–144

27. Vernon CC, Hand JW, Field SB et al (1996) Radiotherapy with or without hyperthermia in the treatment of superficial localized breast cancer: results from five randomized controlled trials—International Collaborative Hyperthermia Group. Int J Radiat Oncol Biol Phys 35: 731–744
28. Zagar TM, Vujaskovic Z, Formenti S et al (2014) Two phase I dose-escalation/pharmacokinetics studies of low temperature liposomal doxorubicin (LTLD) and mild local hyperthermia in heavily pretreated patients with local regionally recurrent breast cancer. Int J Hyperthermia 30(5):285–294
29. Mallory M, Gogineni E, Jones GC et al (2016) Therapeutic hyperthermia: the old, the new, and the upcoming. Crit Rev Oncol Hematol 97:56–64
30. Hurwitz M, Stauffer P et al (2014) Hyperthermia, radiation and chemotherapy: the role of heat in multidisciplinary cancer care. Semin Oncol 41(6):714–729
31. Datta NR, Ordóñez SG, Gaipl US et al (2015) Local hyperthermia combined with radiotherapy and-/or chemotherapy: recent advances and promises for the future. Cancer Treat Rev 41(9):742–753
32. Wust P, Hildebrandt B, Sreenivasa G et al (2002) Hyperthermia in combined treatment of cancer. Lancet Oncol 3(8):487–497, Review
33. Maluta S, Kolff MW (2015) Role of hyperthermia in breast cancer locoregional recurrence: a review. Breast Care (Basel) 10(6):408–412
34. Samulski TV, Grant WJ, Oleson JR et al (1990) Clinical experience with a multi-element ultrasonic hyperthermia system: analysis of treatment temperatures. Int J Hyperthermia 6(5):909–922
35. Myerson RJ, Moros EG, Diederich CJ et al (2014) Components of a hyperthermia clinic: recommendations for staffing, equipment, and treatment monitoring. Int J Hyperthermia 30(1):1–5
36. Oldenborg S, Griesdoorn V, van Os R et al (2015) Reirradiation and hyperthermia for irresectable locoregional recurrent breast cancer in previously irradiated area: size matters. Radiother Oncol 117(2):223–228

The manufacturer's authorised representative in the EU is Springer
Nature Customer Service Centre GmbH, Europaplatz 3, 69115 Heidelberg,
Germany. If you have any concerns regarding our products, please
contact ProductSafety@springernature.com

Printed and bound by CPI Group (UK) Ltd, Croydon, CR0 4YY
27/04/2026
02097623-0001